I0420787

One
Mouthful
at a time

One *Mouthful* at a time

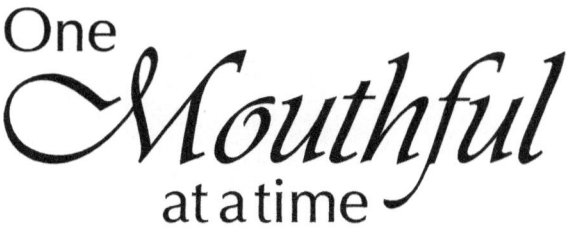

SUTRAS FOR EATING

MYRA KLOCKENBRINK

© 2012 by Myra Klockenbrink
All rights reserved.
ISBN 978-1-300-37037-6

For Steve who — no matter where I travel,
how far I go — is there, always, waiting for me

"*Food is a meditation, a sadhana and a prayer. Good food is a virtue. Food can change your attitude, your behavior, your future, your present. It can change your health, wealth, happiness, everything.*"

—Siri Singh Sahib

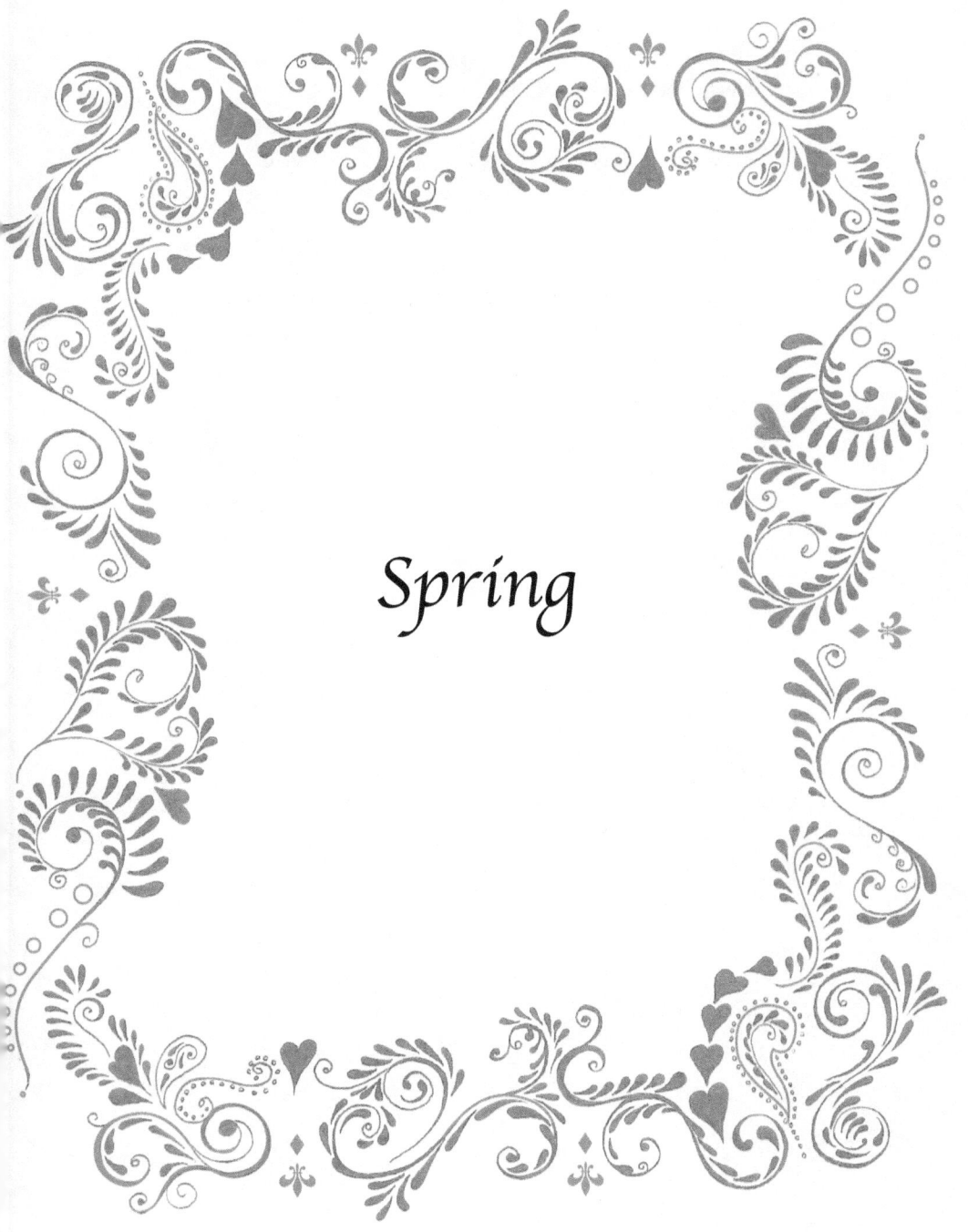

Spring

Drinking Water

Upon rising drink a glass of water (8-12 ounces.) Later with breakfast sip another glass.

Between breakfast and lunch, drink a glass of water. Again, just before lunch, drink another. With lunch sip one more glass.

Between lunch and supper drink a glass of water. Again, before supper, have another glass. With supper sip one more glass.

Between supper and bedtime, drink a glass of water.

OUR BEGINNINGS

At Hell's Gate the river is jumping
waves boil and the white water
is so many moving maws
  full of greedy teeth
    opening and snapping shut

The tide drives the river up its own throat
  it heaves high and heavy
  retching it makes its turn
then smooths the river as flat as a table cloth

The river's special pulse rings our islands
  tugs at our rhythms
  talks to us as the water in us
slaps smartly up against the wall of our every cell

Water is the handmaiden of our happiness:
  in the dew that wets the grass
  in the work that whets our thirst

You need only to see it wrinkle and bubble
  the light in morning to know joy
Beauty is but a bow into the ocean
  to cleave the brine of our beginnings

If ever you have doubt or feel
  you may be stepping awry
or if you are too tired to think
  too stuck in your own head
go and counsel with the water —

  Drink water and experience gratitude

Drink deeply
think no thoughts
allow the water to put you right

Cod Cakes

MAKES 8 CAKES

3 tablespoons coconut oil
1 yellow onion, finely chopped
1 pound cod fillet, bones removed
2 tablespoons parsley, finely minced
1 egg, lightly beaten
Pinch of cayenne pepper
½ cup corn meal
½ cup flour
Salt and freshly ground pepper

Heat olive oil in skillet over medium heat. Add onion and cook until translucent. Set aside.

Cut fish into large chunks; pulse in a food processor into a course chop. Transfer to a medium bowl. Add onion, herbs, egg and cayenne. Mix thoroughly. Add ½ teapoon salt and pepper.

Combine cornmeal, flour, ½ teaspoon salt and ¼ teaspoon pepper. Form 8 3-inch patties with fish and dredge in cornmeal mixture. Heat 1 tablespoon oil in each of two skillets over medium-low heat. Cook 4 patties in each skillet until brown, about 4 minutes on each side.

Serve immediately with a sauce made from the following ingredients, combined well in a small bowl.

Tartar Sauce

1/3 cup mayonnaise
1 tablespoon of dijon mustard
2 teaspoons capers, chopped
1 teaspoon lemon juice
1 tablespoon parsley or dill, minced
Salt and jarred horseradish to taste

THE FOURTH MEAL

In the afternoon of late winter
the sun paints the buildings
in bright light and deep shadow
children scamp and shout
their eyes spark and shine oblivious
to the cold still sharp
and keen to lesser souls

These same children come in
stamping and steaming
  hungry as horses
For times like these forks are too fussy:
  snacks are food we eat with our hands

Cod run through the food processor
salted and formed into small cakes might answer
dredge in cornmeal
fry in good oil, coconut smells wonderful
until they crisp on each side
opalescent in the middle

Have the children dip the fish
in a sauce made with mayonnaise, dijon,
horseradish, capers, lemon juice and dill
the tang will match their appetites
and the fish will eat their hunger

Soufflé

SERVES 6

3 tablespoons butter, softened
Grated Parmesan cheese
12 shallots, minced
4 tablespoons flour
1 cup milk
Pinch of ground nutmeg
Salt and freshly ground pepper to taste
Pinch of cayenne pepper
1 cup Gruyère cheese, grated
4 egg yolks
6 egg whites
Pinch of cream of tartar

Heat oven to 400°. Butter soufflé dish and dust with cheese.

Cut a collar from parchment paper to wrap the dish and to extend 3 inches above rim. Butter inside of collar and tie around dish using kitchen string. Chill the dish.

In a medium saucepan sauté shallots in butter over medium heat until translucent. Add flour and cook for 3 minutes. Add milk, nutmeg, salt and pepper and cayenne. Sit until smooth.

Bring to a brief boil, lower heat and simmer gently for 5 minutes, stirring constantly. Add cheese and stir until incorporated. Mixture should be well-seasoned. Stir in yolks one at a time.

In a large bowl beat egg whites with cream of tartar until stiff and glossy. Mix one cup of the whites into the

STAVING OFF DESPAIR

It's about now that we start to flag
so near the end of winter yet
in her last bitter throes
we begin to lose our resolve

Now is when you have to
make your best effort:
summon all that you are
rise to the occasion
do something grand – make a soufflé

Heat your oven to 400°
butter the inside of a soufflé dish
coat it with grated parmesan cheese
keep it in the fridge while you work the rest
you'll need a half dozen eggs separated
hold each cool mass in your hand until
all that's left is the plump yolk
Keep going
melt a couple tablespoons butter
whisk in a quarter cup flour until it thickens
now add in a half cup milk and whisk that smooth
add salt, pepper, some grated nutmeg, cayenne
scrape it all into a bowl
whisk in the yolks one at a time
to that add your choice of cheese, aged goat is nice

Now stir in a big spoonful of spun egg whites
fold in the rest
pour into your cold soufflé dish
pop into the hot oven and bake for 30 minutes

See how pretty it is

cheese mixture. Fold in remaining egg whites gently into cheese mixture. Pour into chilled soufflé dish.

Bake in lower third of oven for 15 minutes. Reduce heat to 375° and continue to bake for 15 more minutes. Remove collar and serve immediately.

If at a moment of effort
you find it too much
look at a plant, a tree
meditate on their quiet grace
and an ease will come to you
Imitate, imitate
be like a tree, a new leaf, a flower bud
holding itself just so
against every probability

Bone Soup

MAKES 6 CUPS

Stock

5 pounds beef bones
2 carrots, roughly chopped
1 celery stalk
1 onion, cut into quarters, skin on
1 bay leaf
Salt and freshly ground pepper

Cover bones with water in a stock pot and bring to a boil over high heat. Lower heat to a simmer and cook for one hour, skimming fat and foam from surface.

Add vegetables, 2 teaspoons salt, 1 teaspoon pepper and 2 quarts cold water. Simmer for another 2 hours.

Strain stock through a fine sieve. Refrigerate until the fat has congealed sufficiently on the top to remove it.

Soup

6 cups beef stock
1 cup dried navy beans
1/3 cup barley kernels, hulled
2 stalks celery, diced small
2 small leeks, chopped fine
½ teaspoon dried thyme
Salt and freshly ground pepper
1 carrot, diced small
½ cup cabbage, finely chopped
½ cup kale leaves, finely chopped
3 tablespoons parsley, minced

Place stock, beans and barley in a medium pot with the celery, leeks, thyme and 1 teaspoon salt and pepper to taste. Cook at a simmer for 35 minutes. Add carrot, cabbage and kale and cook for another 15 minutes. Check seasonings. Stir in the parsley. Serve.

WHAT IT IS TO BE A TREE

A tree, called a sycamore,
sweeps above the black trestle,
its bark mottled white,
its trunk muscular no less
majestic than the Empire State
in the distance behind it
Chain-link and tires are garbled beneath it
a plastic bag waves spastically from branches
deeply articulated and filled
with crenelated balls of seed

The higher sun has stirred
the wind's whisper of spring
driving scent from the surrounding pines
and perfuming the air momentarily with heat

The wind pushes on, scours the sky
and scatters the seed balls,
leaves them dismantled and cornered in our gutters —
each mote pronged with a sharp claw
a digger to cleave the black earth

Spring may be in the wings
but we are still on stage with winter
and bone soup cooked with leeks, celery,
barley and beans is what we want and need
Cover the beans with bone broth
Add a handful of barley kernels
Cook until the beans are just tender
then add salt, black pepper, a carrot,
pretty cabbage and a few leafy greens
Cook some more, not long

The seed, hard as a nail, has no agenda — it's simply a seed
It waits a timeless time to become a man
standing as a sycamore — in a forest of other men

Vegetables with Yogurt Dip

MAKES 6 SERVINGS

1 pound assorted vegetables, such as cauliflower,
   carrots, broccoli, snap peas, cut into bite-sized
   pieces
1 red pepper, seeded and cut lengthwise into
   ½-inch slices
4 celery stalks, cut into 3" lengths
15 grape tomatoes, halved
Salt

Prepare an ice bath in a medium-sized bowl. Place
steamer basket in medium pan and add 2 cups of
water and 1 teaspoon salt. Make sure the water
does not submerge the bottom of the basket. Place
assorted vegetables in steamer basket and bring water
to a boil. Steam for 2 minutes. Remove from heat,
drain and place vegetables in an ice bath. When they
have cooled completely, drain and pat dry.

Arrange steamed vegetables, red pepper, celery and
tomato halves on a platter. Serve with yogurt dip.

Yogurt Dip

MAKES 1½ CUPS

1 cup whole milk yogurt
1 clove garlic
½ cup fresh herbs, such as parsley, dill,
   cilantro and tarragon, finely minced
10 leaves mint, finely minced
1 tablespoon lemon juice
½ teaspoon salt
¼ teaspoon freshly ground pepper

Strain yogurt through a fine sieve over a small bowl.
When the yogurt has been drained of its whey and
is thick, scrape into a clean bowl. Stir in garlic, herbs,
lemon juice, salt and pepper.

OPPORTUNITIES

In the early
   part of morning
with the first few breaths
 of the new
    day I hear
no thing

The birds have yet
   to sing in the light
It's only me,
   the sleeping,
and the neighbor across the trees
   who never extinguishes her lamp

I am aware
   but not completely awake
no demands are made
   of me

I let what thoughts I have
   float past like clouds
my person-hood and all
   it represents is allowed
to be simply
   interesting
      and inconsequential

I sit and breathe
   like a rock
that soaks up the heat
   of the sun

Crack!

A clear crack parts the silence —

It comes from the spray of daffodils
   not fully opened in their vase

The buds wrapped in paper sheaths
   crack
      open
         under the push of the flower

Here it is:
   Spring

Take the whole day
   and eat nothing
      but vegetables:
raw with a dip of yogurt, garlic and fresh herbs,
lightly steamed with lemon,
sautéed in a pan with ginger,
juiced into an elixir

This is your opportunity
   the door is open
      wide

You can walk right in

Chicken Broth

MAKES 3 QUARTS

2 pounds chicken bones
6 chicken thighs with bone in
2 carrots, cut into large dice
2 celery stalks, cut into large dice
2 leeks with leaves, cleaned and cut into large dice
1 yellow onion, quartered with skin on
¼ teaspoon black peppercorns
2 teaspoons salt
1 teaspoon thyme
½ bunch parsley

Place chicken in stock pot, cover with 4 quarts water
and bring to a boil. Simmer 20 minutes, skimming
off foam and fat from the surface of the broth as
needed. Remove thighs, pull off meat and reserve in
refrigerator. Return bones to broth.

Add remaining ingredients. Bring to a boil. Reduce heat
to the slightest simmer and cover. Continue to simmer
12 hours and up to 24 hours.

Remove from heat and pour stock through fine sieve
into a large bowl. Discard solids. Refrigerate stock until
fat congeals on the surface. Remove excess fat with a
spoon.

Use stock immediately or store in refrigerator for up
to 3 days. Stock can be frozen in quart containers for
up to 3 months.

GOOD COMPANY

Saturday night before the movie
put a chicken in a pot
cover with cold water
and then some

add two carrots
two stalks celery
and an onion

bring to a boil
lower the flame and
skim the foam from the top
keep at an oh-so-slight simmer

Sunday night at dinner time
turn off the heat

ladle the potful through a fine sieve
stir in a bunch minced parsley

Refrigerate the stock
spoon off the fat
use the broth to nourish you and yours
in soups consomme, maybe risotto
use the fat to cook something else

buy the best chicken you can find
one that has lived under the sun
with its feet in the grass

thank the chicken thank yourself
  good food
    good company

Cleansing Broth

MAKES 1 CUP

1 cup water, boiling hot
1 teaspoon tamari sauce
½ teaspoon lemon juice, freshly squeezed
Scant pinch cayenne pepper
½ teaspoon scallion greens, minced

Put all ingredients in a cup. Add hot water. Serve.

THE DREAM

Today the trees are limned in white light
up-lit by some unnamed source
    below ground
at a glance they give
    the spring scene a blurred indistinct glow

In a matter of days they will end
    their silence
bud by bud their light will turn
into a cacophony of color and scent
    and our world will be transformed

Don't disturb the dream
by eating too much
a light broth made with hot water
from the kettle and enough tamari sauce
to offset a fat squeeze of lemon juice
a few grains of cayenne and
a mincing of scallion greens
might be all it takes to ease an appetite

Let the energy of the season bubble up
    through you
feed it lightly and water it well
    Find the sun and welcome it back

Spring Salad
MAKES 4 CUPS

1 small bunch arugula, rinsed, trimmed of stems,
    torn into small pieces
10 stems dandelion leaves, rinsed, trimmed of
    stems, torn into small pieces
1 small bunch watercress, rinsed, trimmed of
    stems, torn into small pieces
½ cup fresh herbs such as parsley, tarragon, dill and
    chives, rinsed, trimmed of stems and minced
1 grapefruit, peeled and supremed, reserving juice

Dressing
MAKES 1 CUP

½ cup olive oil
¼ cup balsamic vinegar
1 tablespoon dijon mustard
2 tablespoons pepitas, ground
½ teaspoon salt
¼ teaspoon pepper freshly ground

Combine salad ingredients in large bowl, including juice
from grapefruit. Toss with dressing as desired. Serve
immediately.

ALL WE NEED

All we need
is at our feet
we have but to pick it up

The trees are stuffed with flowers
their petals swirl around us
        a wistful confetti
the new leaves drape the branches
like so many newborn butterflies

Our bodies crave to take part
without compunction we begin to build salads
deep greens like arugula, dandelion and
the watercress that is springing up in our creeks
add a fat handful of fresh herbs:
        parsley, tarragon, chives, dill
strip a pink grapefruit of its membranes
right over the bowl

Now whisk together some ground pumpkin seeds
a little balsamic vinegar, dijon and
of course olive oil
dress your salad with your hands
there's no harm in it

Step out into the gentle day
it offers you peace
        in its upturned hand
take it and carry it in your heart

        You won't regret it

Avocado Hair Mask

MAKES 1 CUP

1 ripe avocado
1 egg yolk
1 tablespoon honey

Scoop the avocado from its skin and mash into a small bowl. Add egg yolk and whip into avocado until well-mixed. Add honey. Stir until smooth.

Apply first to scalp with dry hair. Work the mixture into the hair all the way to the bottom of the strands, until all the hair is covered

Wrap long hair around head, then cover with a 2-foot length of plastic wrapped tightly around your head.

Take a small-sized bath towel, wet and squeeze dry. Fold into quarters and microwave for 30-second intervals until towel is hot, but not too hot to handle.

Unfold and wrap towel around your head. When towel cools repeat once or twice for a total wrap time of about 20 minutes.

Rinse hair completely. Shampoo. The treatment acts as the conditioner.

WHILE WE SLEPT

Overnight it snowed
   sugaring the grass
and I was oblivious in sleep
in the morning it shone pink
   in the day's new light

I didn't see the forsythia bloom either
   but there it is
lighting up bedraggled gardens

And if you look up the street
   you'll see how the trees have filled out
creating a haze of potentiality

The Big Dipper has pushed Orion offstage
   the bluebird has already built its nest
   and calves romp in the warming light

Where was I when all this happened?
   Dreaming it in?

The season is unpacking
   it comes without our seeing it
yet surrounds and enfolds us
becomes us - behold it
let spring see itself
   how ravishing it is

Take care of yourself
   tend to your body:
Blend some avocado with an egg
   yolk and rub it into your hair
wind plastic wrap around your head
   and a hot towel after that
Look out the window —
   something amazing is happening there

Rice with Herbs

MAKES 4 SERVINGS

1 cup brown basmati rice, soaked overnight in
    water with 1 teaspon lemon juice
1 cup fresh peas, shelled
½ cup parsley, minced
¼ cup tarragon, minced
zest of one lemon
Salt and freshly ground black pepper

Bring 2 cups water to a boil with ½ teaspoon salt.
Rinse rice. Add to boiling water with parsley and
tarragon and cover. Lower heat to a simmer and
cook for 20 minutes or until all the water has been
absorbed. Remove from heat, cover and allow to rest
10 minutes.

Prepare an ice bath in a medium-sized bowl. Place
steamer basket in small pan and add 2 cups of water
and ¼ teaspoon salt. Make sure the water does not
submerge the bottom of the basket. Place peas in
steamer basket and bring water to a boil. Steam for 2
minutes. Remove from heat, drain and place peas in an
ice bath. When they have cooled completely, drain and
pat dry.

In a large bowl gently fold peas into rice with the
lemon zest and ½ teaspoon pepper. Check seasonings.
Serve.

THE BEES

The buds of the early cherries look shellacked —
glossy beads erupt with papery pink petals that push
themselves out into the blue
and delicately expose their sex parts

The woolly bees come and rumple these tumescent filaments
they hump the blossoms for all they are worth —
  first this one, then another
  no, not that one
  oh! this one is gooood

The flowers have no leaves to cover them
they have no shame, no hesitation,
no mind to soil their perfection

In a few days, tomorrow maybe,
the rain or wind will have the petals
They'll leave behind their sex fulfilled
and without our knowing, seeing or realizing
the ripe fruit will fill the trees
to dangle down in the shade of the leaves

This new weather drives us from our kitchens
and lightens our appetites
steamed brown rice will suffice
that and a fat handful of minced fresh herb —
parsley and tarragon are nice —
with shelled sweet peas

Take your bowl outside
see if you can catch a glimpse
of the quiet riot in the trees

Crème Fraîche

MAKES I CUP

I cup heavy cream
2 tablespoons buttermilk

Combine cream and buttermilk in a small jar. Stir until well blended. Let stand at room temperature for 24 hours or until thickened. Refrigerate to store.

FREE LOVE

The baby train came down the walk this morning
six, eight! babies propped in a wagon
like new loaves of bread
   or fresh sacks of milk
      ready to be delivered
the morning sun glittering in their hair

   They rocked in their wagon
   passing out handfuls of free love
   to anyone who would take it

Even the dogs
   especially the dogs
smiled when they passed
the big one slapped his tail
back and forth with a happy thud
the little one licked at the babies' toes

Small wonder —
they sat fat and alert
the creases in their arms
and under their chins
like thick cream piled up on cake

Now that the weather's warm
you can make your own
tangy cream fraiche — a rich sour cream:
pour a couple tablespoons of buttermilk
into a pint carton full of heavy cream
give it a shake and let it set for a day
until the cream thickens

It's good dolloped over most anything:
strawberries, of course

borscht, spicy tacos
warm chocolate cake

The babies' job is to drink milk and grow
Our job is to feel the sun warm our backs
to cradle our own goodness and serve it up —
    pluck away anxiety, doubt, bitterness —
worry never brought anything good into the world

Abandon your cares
    and take up your best self
    dandle it in your lap

Give yourself over
    to all who pass

Dandelion Beet Salad

MAKES 2 SERVINGS

2 tablespoons bacon fat
    (olive oil is a fine substitute)
2 cups dandelion leaves, rinsed, stems removed,
    torn into small pieces
1 medium beet, peeled and cut in 2-inch long
    ¼-inch thick sticks
1 small sweet onion, sliced into ½-inch strips
Salt and freshly ground pepper
1 tablespoon raspberry vinegar

Heat fat in medium sauté pan over medium heat. Add onions and beets and stir until coated in fat cooking gently for 2 minutes. Add rinsed and wet dandelion leaves and salt to taste. Lower heat and cover, cooking for five minutes or until beets are tender, adding a teaspoon or two of water as necessary.

Remove from heat. Add pepper to taste and vinegar. Toss well. Serve.

WINTER IS GONE

Winter is gone
celebrate and find a nearby field
step lightly — the earth is tender
notice all the life pushing up out of the ground
soon you will see a dandelion
then another — more
See how they look:
like they have been shoved up through a funnel
how their blossoms open in the morning sun
The flowers are good to eat
but that's a different story

Pluck the serrated leaves
until you have a fat handful

At home rinse them well and chop them up
take a beet, peel and cube it

In some olive oil cook
thinly sliced onion
shallots are good here too
saute them until they glisten
add the beets, a few spoons of water and a lid
steam until the beets are just tender
toss in the dandelions and salt
cook until the broth has left and the greens are vibrant

Now splash with some good vinegar–
raspberry! is lovely here

Congratulate yourself
It is spring in the twenty-first century
you have touched the ground
and eaten from it —
      a noble deed you will not forget

Carrots & Rice
MAKES TWO SERVINGS

1 cup short grain brown rice
Lemon juice
1 tablespoon butter
½ teaspoon salt
1 carrot, cut in ¼-inch dice
¼ cup Vidalia onion, chopped fine
½ cup peas, shelled
1 tablespoon mint, minced
Freshly ground pepper

Soak rice covered with water with a squeeze of lemon juice for at least 2 hours or overnight. Drain and rinse.

Bring 2 cups of water to a boil in a medium-sized pot. Add rice, butter and salt. Reduce heat to low and cover. Cook for 30 minutes.

Lay carrot, onion and peas over rice. Cover and cook another 15 minutes.

Remove from heat. Add mint and replace cover. Allow to sit for 10 minutes. Fluff rice gently with pepper to taste.

PLENTY

There is enough in the flowers
    in the shadows of the new leaves
There is enough in my child's face
    listening to music
There is enough brilliance in the sun
    freshness in the shade
There is enough in the man with a cane
    reading the newspaper
There is enough in the birds' chattering calls
    their quick matings in the trees

There is enough food in a pot of brown rice
    steamed with carrots & onions sliced fine
    to feed you and your kin at midday
There are enough complexities to rampage the earth
   simple food is not one of them

There is enough
    we have enough

Ginger Tea

2-inch length ginger root
1 teaspoon lemon juice
scant pinch cayenne pepper
2 teaspoons honey

Peel ginger root with the side of a spoon. Slice very thin and place in a small pan filled with 2 cups water. Bring to a boil, reduce heat and simmer over low heat for 10 minutes. Strain.

Place lemon juice, cayenne and honey in a cup. Pour ginger tea over all and stir.

THIS LIGHT

Dawn comes in
through the one open window
    and spills onto the floor
It bathes the children
mindlessly sleeping in their beds
and reaches us as we sit
    in the great unfolding quiet

This light which took so long
    to reach us
greens the trees
turns the faces of the flowers
and sets the birds to singing
It brightens the clouds
and casts their shadows
over the receiving landscape.

This light brings out the colors
that make this wall bright
that wall dark,
rings this thing we call a cup in shining white
and prompts the great wheel of our activity

But before we begin we can honor our meeting with the light
with a simple tea made from fresh ginger and lemon
nothing complicated — just good

We have traveled our life long
to get to this point
    this moment our destination
our rendezvous with this light

Nothing more than a moment ourselves
in the life of the light
and yet it shines on us as if we alone
    were meant to receive it

Grill-Style Artichokes

MAKES 2 SERVINGS

1 artichoke
1 teaspoon coconut oil
1 lemon
2 tablespoons butter
Salt and freshly ground pepper

Snip the leaf points from the artichoke with a pair of kitchen shears. Cut the artichoke in half lengthwise. Scoop out the thistle-like choke using a melon baller or spoon.

Heat oil in cast iron skillet large enough to hold both artichoke halves over medium heat. Place artichokes face down on the hot skillet and cover.

Cook for 12-15 minutes depending on the size of the artichoke. A knife should easily pierce the artichoke all the way through.

Serve with lemon butter.

Lemon Butter

Melt the butter in a small saucepan over low heat. When the milk solids have gathered at the bottom of the pan, carefully scrap off the foam from the surface of the butter. Slowly pour into a small bowl, leaving the milk solids behind in the pan.

Add 2 teaspoons lemon juice to the butter. Salt to taste.

NOISE

Before it is morning
  when the sun is still
  rolling over the Atlantic Ocean
  and it is midnight in Japan
    it is very quiet
    very easy to sit in silence
We are still
  halfway between dreams
  and daytime dramas
  we can listen carefully
  to the clear ring of no sound

Until as the light turns
  and begins to take on color
  the garbage truck rolls up the street
  chuffing and braking
  the men's voices as they call
  to one another a clarion
  of the brightening light

The birds pitch in
  each pressing their own key
  repeat repeat repeat
  the garbage truck leads the parade
  cars line up behind it
  some old metal cabinet
  now being fitted into its maw

Still the silence rings
  holding the truck, the humming cars,
  the repeating birds
  and the scratch of the pen across the paper

For a time no-sound sounds
  and there is nothing
  only this breath

and before another is taken
there is that nothing again
that short, eternal, pause
and from that bottomless cup
   everything else blooms

Artichokes are on the shelves now
find a tight heavy head and bring it home
trim away the sharp spines and cut it in half lengthwise
scoop out the prickly choke with a spoon

Heat a cast iron skillet and glaze it with a coin of oil
place the artichoke halves face-down
and a lid on the pan

At medium-low heat the artichoke will cook
steamed in its own moisture
its face slightly charred

It's hard to beat salted lemon juice
and melted butter for dipping the leaves
one by one until you reach the tender heart
the prize for your patience

The morning advances at full tilt
   empty garbage cans strewn in its wake
The light is entwined to the lowest reaches of the trees
   and the people press purposefully within it
A new day is launched — a new expression
   from the surrounding silence

We have not always been ready
   to hear the silence sound
   beneath the ruckus of life

But more and more we can hear it
   and recognize it issues from within
      our beating heart

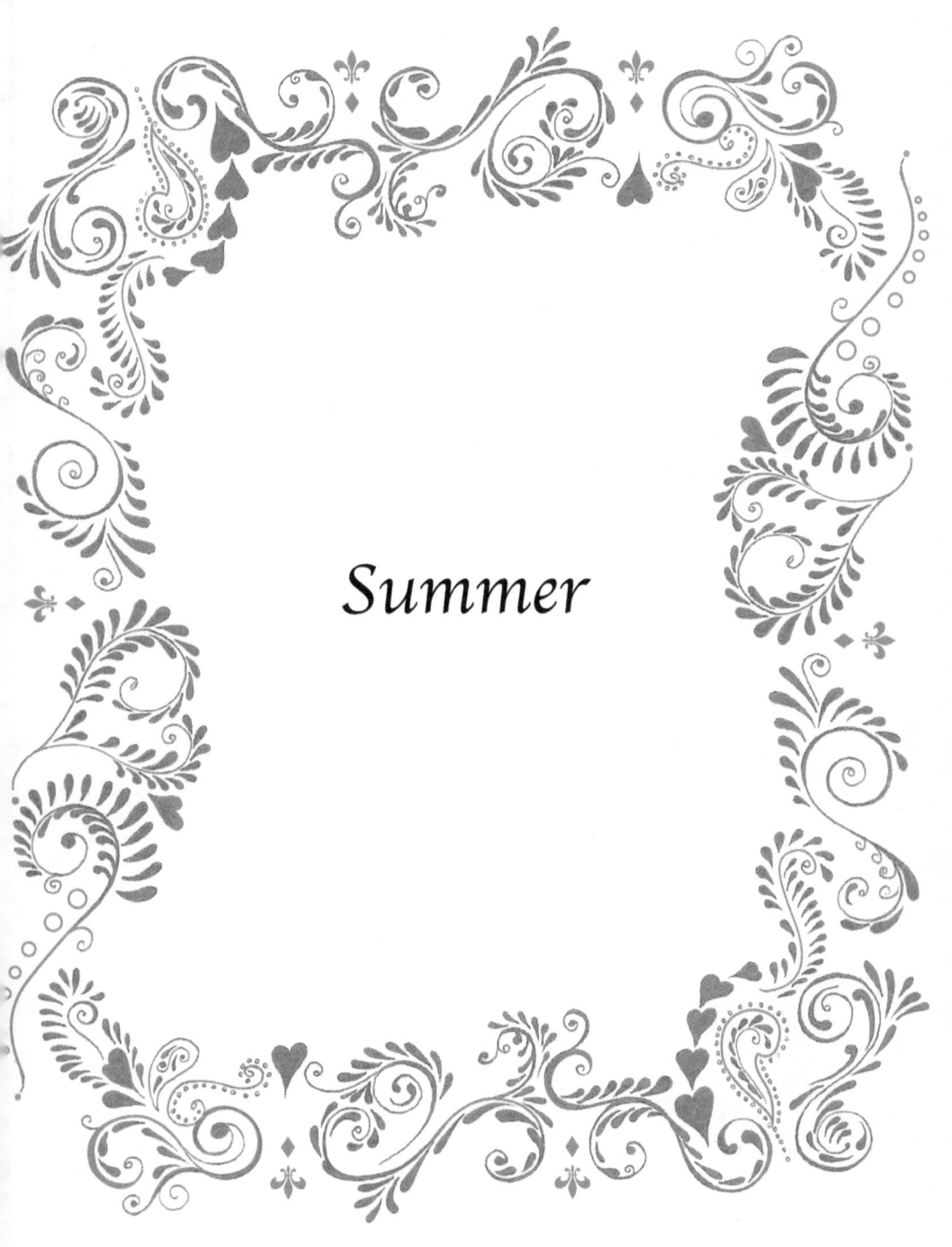

Summer

Tea Drink
MAKES 2 QUARTS

1 heaping tablespoon dried peppermint leaves
1 heaping tablespoon dried rose hips
1 heaping tablespoon dried chamomile
1 heaping tablespoon rooibos leaves
1 teaspoon dried hibiscus leaves
1 teaspoon dried stevia leaves

Place herbs in a glass pitcher and pour 1 quart of boiling water over all. Cover and allow to cool.

Strain tea through a fine mesh strainer. Return to pitcher and add 1 quart cold water. Refrigerate.

WITCHCRAFT

The sun's pass across the sky
takes longer now
warming the earth
sending the people out
with the other animals
to enjoy the cool night air

It's getting hot!

We need something to drink
a concoction of equal parts
mint, rose hips, chamomile, rooibos
a fat tablespoon of each
and less of hibiscus – a teaspoon maybe

Pour a quart of boiling water over all
in a glass pitcher and let the plants
yield their magic until the tea is dark and red
strain out the herbs and
add another quart of cool water

It's good warm
refreshing cold

A spoon of stevia leaf when it steeps
will sweeten it, but doesn't need it

Be undaunted
these gentle plants are there
look a little and you'll find them

Sounds like witchcraft — it is
drink it up
give it to your children
make everybody happy
  then do it again tomorrow

Rhubarb Tea

MAKES 2 QUARTS

8 cups rhubarb stalks, cut into 2-inch lengths
¼ cup agave nectar

Place rhubarb and 2 quarts water in a large pan. Cover.
Bring to a simmer. Cook for one hour. Allow to cool.

Strain through a fine sieve into a glass pitcher. Stir in
agave nectar. Refrigerate before serving.

BUT ONCE

The thicket is in
what's left of negative space
has been relegated to the sky
   and the latticework of treetops

Every shade of green is represented
to look upon it all
is to somehow know that
green is the color of wellness

Rhubarb has pushed up its red stalks
and that improbable large green leaf
now's your chance:
some door's open but once and briefly

Go on, make some punch
one stalk rhubarb to one cup of water
cut it into finger lengths
and simmer in a covered pot,
for about an hour

This way it yields
its natural refreshing sweetness
a spoon of agave nectar is all you'll need
to get it just right

Get your exercise
then sit back and put up your feet
and have a glass of this lovely pink nonpareil

Watch the wind carry the summer in
and how the greenery, unflustered,
   beckons

Early Summer Salad
MAKES 2 SERVINGS

4 cups wild greens, such as chickweed, lambs quarters,
    dandelion, violet leaves and young greens, such as
    kale, arugula, and lettuces.
½ cup violet and cherry blossoms

Soak greens in cold water to clean several times if
necessary. Drain. Spin dry in a salad spinner.

Dress with vinaigrette. Add flower blossoms to bowl.
Serve immediately.

Vinaigrette Dressing
MAKES I CUP

I cup olive oil
¼ cup white wine vinegar
2 tablespoons lemon juice
I tablespoons onion grass or chives, minced
I tablespoon Dijon mustard
3/4 teaspoon salt
½ teaspoon freshly ground pepper

Mix all the ingredients in a jar with a tight-fitting lid.
Shake well until completely emulsified. Refrigerate to
store.

DOMESTIC WEEDS

The moment you take yourself
to the garden and begin to dig
a deep peace descends
To-do thoughts stop crowding
and the moment blooms
    into a surrounding calm

The soil feels warm
a black blanket for the seeds
We're planting now - at the Farm
the weeds gleam green
that tender green splendor
a deep rain produces:
chickweed, lambs quarters, dandelion
volunteers from last year:
arugula, kale, lettuces

A pity to till them under
when in their wildness they nourish as no crop can
Before you plant your peas, tomatoes
your herbs and cabbages
snip these feral plantlets into your basket
    and make a salad

Be sure to include the odd violet blossom
  the cherry blossom petals spangling the dirt
Dress this bounty with half each lemon juice
and wine vinegar to two parts olive oil (a little math)
add good mustard, salt, black pepper
and a fat dose of minced onion grass - rife now
With some goats milk cheese,
sunflower seeds and crusty bread
    you can toast your garden —
    the one you never had to plant
    the one to come
        and all things wild

Watercress and Sardines
MAKES 2 SERVINGS

2 cups watercress leaves, stems removed
1 4.25-ounce can of sardines, packed in oil
2 eggs, hard-boiled and peeled

Soak watercress in cold water. Drain. Spin dry in salad spinner. Place in large bowl. Dress with yogurt dressing and toss.

Drain sardines of their oil. Crumble onto watercress.

Slice eggs into quarters. Add to salad. Serve.

Yogurt Dressing
MAKES 1 CUP

½ cup whole milk yogurt
¼ cup mayonnaise
1 tablespoon lemon juice
1 small clove garlic, minced
2 tablespoons tarragon, minced
Salt and freshly ground pepper

Blend yogurt, mayonnaise and lemon juice in a small bowl. Add garlic, tarragon, ½ teaspoon salt and ¼ teaspoon pepper.

Stir well. Refrigerate to store.

KNOWING

In the late evening
the sky is full of light
though the sun traveled on
more than an hour ago

There wrapped in her nest
a bluebird sleeps curled over her chicks
the nest radiates a deep warmth
    her iridescent feathers shining
From them the night sky spills
with its blaze of stars
and her eye gleams black with wild mystery

The air is scented sweet and cool
the fireflies have lit their lamps
and the trees fringe the coloring sky
with their black branches

The evening offers up its perfection
we move through it like the beasts of the sea
it is our medium down to the last unseen detail:
the particles spinning in their ether
the moon yet to rise
the gentle tilt of the earth
    poised on her axis

We stroll through the grass to dinner
watercress fills the cold streams and is in flower
the bunched tips make a flavorful salad
topped with chopped hard-cooked eggs
and crumbled sardines
a tangy dressing made with yogurt
mayonnaise, lemon juice, garlic, tarragon and salt
is the perfect counterpoint to this spicy green

The evening deepens
the sky replete with stars
it would seem they have descended
to frolic in the grass
and dance among the tree tops
flying as they do with their small lamps of fire

The bluebird in her nest is a fact
but this knowledge says nothing
    of her heat and light
    in the darkness
how her black eyes shine
with everything we do not know
    yet recognize within ourselves
the way the deepening evening light
    knows the dark charge of night

Grilled Apricots

SERVES 4

8 ripe apricots, washed, patted dry, cut in half and pitted
1 tablespoon unsalted butter
¼ cup cane juice crystals or coconut sugar
1¼ cups whole milk yogurt
¼ cup chopped pistachios, toasted

Line a grill rack with aluminum foil. Lay the apricot
halves on the foil, cut side up. Dab each half with a bit
of butter. Sprinkle each half with a ½ teaspoon sugar.

Grill covered for 5 minutes or until the apricots turn
brown at their edges.

Spoon the apricots onto a plate, gathering the juices.
Top each with a tablespoon of yogurt. Sprinkle each with
a teaspoon of nuts.

INSIDE OUTSIDE

Dinner is done
the birds chortle as they settle in
and the squirrels have ceased their scrambling
and gone — where is it they go?
Here and there fireflies signal to one another
incandescent even with the moon shining huge
and improbable over the rooftops

Seize a reason to be outside
invent a cause, fulfill a fantasy
make a profit if you must
  but find a way out

Take your desk to the stoop
shower in the downpours
pull out a mattress
reinstate the constitutional
and walk in the evening
with someone you love
tell them what lies in your heart

It's easy to cook out of doors
after dinner while the grill is still hot
Lay some apricot halves on foil
and dot them with butter and
cane juice crystals

Let them cook until the sugar bubbles
serve them with sheep's milk yogurt
maybe a spoon of granola

You can feel the night grow still
the birds have stopped
the trees themselves seem to rest
Talk about the meaning of this life
now is as good a time as ever

Stone Fruit
MAKES 2 QUARTS

2-4 pounds stone fruit, such as cherries, apricots,
      nectarines, peaches and plums, completely ripe

Bring a large pot of water to boil. Place 2 or 3 of the
same fruit, whole into the boiling water for 30 seconds.
Remove with a slotted spoon. Allow to cool. The skin
should slip from the fruit easily, but the fruit should
remain completely uncooked.

Continue with all the fruit. Cut each fruit into halves,
quarters or slices, depending on its intended use.

Arrange fruit in a jelly roll pan that fits in the freezer
section of your refrigerator. Freeze for 15-30 minutes.

For the cherries, pit cherries with a cherry pitter
before freezing as above.

Store fruit by kind in quart-sized, zip-lock freezer bags
for up to 3 months.

CHORES

The season is working up momentum
the trees have erupted in a dense greenery
To pass under one is a kind of benediction
(it has always been this way
more obvious now in the heat)

The linden exude their perfume in the warm air
catalpas drop their lavish blooms to the ground
open-mouthed, the bees fill the trees and
set them to humming

Farmers work the trees too and bring down their fruits
in quick succession: first cherries
then apricots nectarines peaches and plum

It's almost embarrassing

When you have done your part
and eaten you share on your morning cereal
out-of-hand at lunch and gently poached at dinner
Take the rest, the extra, the impulse five-pound sacks
from the farmers market and freeze them

The cherries you can pit and bag
the other stone fruit gently float
in boiling water for half a minute and cool
slip the fruit from their skins,
slice in wedges and lay
onto a cookie sheet and freeze maybe 15 minutes
then bag them up-they'll stay separate and saved

Until that moment when you are ready to welcome winter
with a gift only the hot sun can bring to bear

It's a homely chore
    but better than money in the bank

Rice Pudding Without the Stove
SERVES 4

2 cups short grain brown rice, cooked
1 cup whole milk yogurt, preferably Bulgarian style
1 tablespoon raw sunflower seeds, hemp o
    ground flax seed
½ cup blueberries
½ teaspoon cinnamon
2 tablespoons maple syrup
¼ cup chopped walnuts, toasted

In a medium bowl mix rice, yogurt, cinnamon and sunflower seeds. Gently fold in blueberries.

Spoon into 4 serving bowls. Drizzle each with a teaspoon or two of maple syrup. Sprinkle with walnuts. Serve.

LISTEN

If you listen beyond
    the thrum of summer sounds
the chime of children in the play yard
beyond the clarion song of birds
the brush of wind through the trees
beyond the hollowing-out sounds of jets and cars
    there is a space of no sound

Hold yourself steady and listen:
    here everything has a bright clarity
an ever-opening calm that holds you
in perfect stillness
    in a space of no time

We go there when we draw, paint, write
whatever the creative act
we can go when we cook —
a perfect place to practice

No need to light the stove
use last night's rice and stir it
into whole milk yogurt
add sunflower seeds, try others
add any or all of the berries
    coming into their season
maybe you like a
drizzle of maple syrup
maybe toasted walnuts
  show me what you like

Go to the place of no time
    at will and often
sit and be steady
watch the tide of your breath
it will take you there —
    the birthplace of happiness

Asian-Style Slaw
SERVES 4

2 cups green cabbage, sliced very fine
1 cup red cabbage, sliced very fine
3 medium-sized plums, rinsed, patted dry, halved,
   pitted, and cut into thin slices
Juice of 2 limes
1½ teaspoons salt
¼ teaspoon chili pepper flakes
½ cup cilantro leaves, roughly chopped
1½ tablespoon toasted sesame oil
½ cup raw cashews

Place cabbage and plums in a large bowl. Using your hands, toss slaw with lime juice and salt, massaging the leaves as you work.

Add pepper flakes, cilantro and sesame oil. Toss well.

Chill for 1 hour.

Serve with cashews sprinkled on top of slaw.

KEEPING TIME

The yellow light slowly slides
down the street
It gilds the trees in patches
and casts bright clouds
over the face of the buildings

Birds jet from branch to branch
  in black streaks interlacing
the quiet with their bright calls

As the air warms it drifts
through the streets
and lifts the leaves of the trees
with a lilting softness

This day in summer is a portrait
  of stillness and ease:
The lily offers its fragrance in its striped cup
The rose reaches ripe and red
  above thorns glinting on its stalk

There's nothing to do
  if there ever was
It's all here — serene and resplendent
with breeze enough to spill
a liquid ring from one clear chime

Dinner now is little more than bending to the earth
  and pulling it up
that and reaching up to the trees
  and shaking it down
A fresh slaw will go with any meal:
cabbage cut fine with plums sliced thin
lime juice, hot pepper flakes, nuts and herbs
all tossed together and served an hour later

60   SUMMER

Join the crowd of life
and ride the undulant wave of summer
see how its pace keeps time
  with your own
    purring pulse

Raspberry Cassis

MAKES 1 QUART

4 cups raspberries
5 tablespoons sugar
3 tablespoons Cassis

Place raspberries in a bowl with sugar and Cassis.
Mix gently.

Chill for 30 minutes before serving.

NOTE: Frozen raspberries can be similarly macerated
at room temperature.

PARTS GREATER THAN THE SUM

Viewed from the forest floor in Colorado
the clotted grey clouds
perfectly offset the green of the trees:
   the short-needled firs stand erect
   alongside the swaying ponderosas and twinkling aspen
together they form a pattern
random, but somehow recognizable
   as is the dispersal of flowers littered among them
   or the lichens spangling the rocks

Deeper through the tangle of undergrowth
a stream rips through the forest
like a crack in the earth letting out the light
   To put your hands into it is to immediately brighten
   The ferocity of its speed over the rocks
   exhilarates all the way to the fear seated in your groin
Its pattern too is familiar
   Though nothing is more random than the spirals it draws
   in its loops and bends down the mountain
   we sense the stillness that lies in its depths and shallows

At camp the children dance around the fire ring
the reaching flames inspire their carousing leaps and song
Like the flames their antics follow no predictable path
but we recognize joy just as we do the fire they feed

   In the kitchen
   a tray of raspberries will form a similar pattern
   so many raspberries — so prone to mold
   But if you place them in a sheet pan
   and give them a good shake
   they will arrange themselves
   away from each other —
   in a clear pattern
      but in no particular order

Once they've frozen hard
they can be packed into freezer bags
and stored without clumping up into a mass
Such a package can be amended
with a little sugar and cassis
and served over pound cake
at the picnic table
an aerated container of pure whipped cream
is easy to transport and the perfect topping
Let the children serve....

Chopped Vegetable Salad With Buttermilk
SERVES 4

4 Persian-style cucumbers, cut lengthwise in
    quarters, then in ½-inch pieces
4 stalks celery, cut in 1-inch lengths
1 green bell pepper, cored and cut into
    1-inch-square pieces
12 red radishes, cut into quarters
¼ cup mint, minced
1 quart buttermilk
2 teaspoons salt
1 teaspoon freshly ground black pepper

Combine all the ingredients in a medium bowl.
Serve immediately.

HUNGER

Rain has made the grass lush
when you lie in it
it accepts all your weight
like a gift and bears you up as if in arms

Look up
the sky looks different from here
with all its clarity, its clouds, its sparkling light
it gives context to all our yearnings

Sit up
have a picnic
children, who have a great sense of occasion,
love picnics
you can eat with your fingers
things like olives, grapes and cheese —
and you don't have to watch where the crumbs fall

Cold buttermilk poured over
diced cucumber, radish, scallion and celery
and dressed with finely chopped mint
good salt and ground pepper
is wonderfully refreshing on a hot day

Everything tastes better more alive
out of doors where we become
especially hungry for some reason
the air, the shimmering pulse of summer
quickens our appetite
and ravenously we talk laugh and play
the grass tickling our feet

Quinoa Pita Pockets
SERVES 6

3/4 cup quinoa, rinsed
3 cups black beans, cooked
Olive oil
1 small yellow onion, chopped fine
3 cloves garlic, minced
1 teaspoon ground cumin
1 teaspoon chili powder
Salt and freshly ground pepper
4 corn on the cob, husked
1 tablespoon butter
1 cup cherry tomatoes, roughly chopped
2 tablespoons cilantro, minced
3 cups mesclun salad greens
Lime wedges
Bottled hot sauce

In a small sauce pan place quinoa, ½ teaspoon salt and
1¼ cup water over high heat. Bring to a boil. Lower
heat, cover and simmer for 20 minutes or until water
has been fully absorbed.

In a small pan, heat 1 tablespoon olive oil. Add onion
and cook over medium-low heat until soft. Add garlic,
cumin and chili powder and continue to cook for
another 3 minutes. Add beans, cover and cook for 10
minutes, adding salt and pepper to taste.

Steam corn in a shallow skillet with one cup of salted
water for 6 minutes. Cool and cut corn from cobs into a
wide shallow bowl to catch kernels. Add butter and stir.

Mix cherry tomatoes and cilantro with juice from one
lime. Add salt and pepper to taste. Wrap pita pockets
in foil. Heat in a 300° oven for 5 minutes before serving.

SATISFACTION

The ocean has no better match
than children playing in her surf
they taunt her jumping and shouting for the big one
here comes the biggest one ever
amidst their squeals monster waves climb
then collapse in a swath of ruffles at their feet

Back and forth they run tireless
as she is and maybe as relentless
when that's done they jump
time again from the lifeguard stand
or dig holes in the sand
until only the tops of their heads peek out

What they bother to eat
often lands in the sand
so pack plenty
pita pockets filled with black beans
quinoa, cheese, some compulsory salad greens
and a squeeze of lime
you can have the freshly made corn kernels,
chopped cherry tomatoes & cilantro in yours
maybe with a little piquant chili sauce
hand-held watermelon triangles will do after

Eating well is no mystery
but what feeds the furious force funneling
through children is beyond
what we know of the moon and the tides
we can be satisfied by the in and out of the seas
but for kids satisfaction is a flat ocean

Corn Soup

SERVES 6

6 ears corn, husked
2 cups chicken stock
2 cups milk
2 tablespoons butter
1 large onion, finely chopped
1 pound waxy potatoes, such as fingerlings
    scrubbed and cut into ½-inch dice
Salt and freshly ground pepper
Pinch cayenne pepper
1 cup heavy cream
½ cup basil, torn into small pieces

Cut kernels from cobs and set aside. Reserve cobs.

In a large saucepan, melt butter over medium-low heat.
Add onion and cook until soft. Add potatoes and corn
kernels and cook for 5 minutes, stirring often.

Add stock, reserved cobs, salt, cayenne and freshly
ground pepper to taste. Turn heat to low and simmer for
20 minutes.

Remove from heat. Remove cobs and discard.

(At this point the mixture can be cooled and pulsed
briefly in the food processor to make creamed corn.
Return mixture to low heat and stir in 1/2 cup of
the heavy cream. Add black pepper to taste and 1
teaspoon sugar. Simmer for 5 minutes until the cream
has thickened. Serve.)

To make the soup add the milk, cream and basil.
Cook for 5 minutes more on low heat. Season to taste
with pepper. Sir and serve.

HOW TO BE A HUMAN BEING

In the early evening
the cattle are driven to a high meadow
birds flit in their wake
pierced by the lowering sun
they are near transparent
    motes in the broad landscape

The cow's gaze is that of a small child:
    honest and open
full of — could it be — tenderness?
Their calves follow with milk-slathered muzzles
and work their way to the soft, downy teats
    at every turn
the mothers are patient though not always
    compliant – backing up
to thwart their babies' persistence

The calves grow fast on all that milk,
which inspires other uses: a cold soup —
diced onions and fresh corn cut from the cob
sauteed with butter in a deep pan
Add diced potatoes, the cobs themselves
a pinch of cayenne and a handful of finely torn basil
Cover with stock, simmering until tender
Cool and with the back of a butter knife
scrape the corn milk from the cobs
then discard them (they compost fine)
The soup can be pureed at this point
  if you're fond of creamed corn
Now add enough whole milk
to get the consistency you like
Season with salt and fresh ground pepper

72   SUMMER

This soup is delicious warm at supper
 refreshing cold at midday

The contract we have with our husbanded animals is sacred
we share the land with them, help them flourish
In return they teach us
 how to be human beings:
 to see them beyond our own needs
 as the relatives they are —
 guardians of our higher selves

Frittata

SERVES 4

2 tablespoons butter
1 large shallot, chopped fine
2 cloves garlic, minced
2 cups lambs quarters, stripped of their stems,
   chopped roughly (Spinach can be substituted.)
8 eggs
Salt and freshly ground pepper to taste
4 ounces goat cheese cut into 1/2'-thick coins
8 artichokes hearts, drained and patted dry

Preheat broiler to medium heat.

Melt butter in well-seasoned cast-iron skillet or nonstick ovenproof pan. Add shallot and garlic and cook over medium heat until translucent. Add lambs quarters. Stir and cook until wilted, about 5 minutes.

Whip eggs with salt and pepper until well-blended and pour into pan. Once the eggs begin to set around the edges of the pan, arrange the artichokes and goat cheese coins on top. Sprinkle with Parmesan cheese. Eggs should still be liquid.

Place under broiler. Cook briefly until the eggs puff and turn golden brown. Remove from oven and immediately slide the frittata onto a cutting board. Cut into wedges and serve.

DAY ONE

The fretted forest offers no order
the pattern, though replete, is random,
chaotic and stymies our willful wanting

Each tree is different
though all of these are shagbark hickories
Each leaf, stem and twig varied
The roots have a common habit
but exercise it differently

Each flower, each thorn, each whorl of lichen
has its own imprint
its own long short life
it plays its own note
for this is the genesis of music

Here and there the trees move in rhythm to it
the oak quivers in the light
each leaf a shining disk
spanking the light back
again and back
until the entire tree glitters
making a sound like grain
running down a sheet metal trough
or like the rain that fell
in the black night to leave mirrors
in every hollow and cup
until the sun burnt them dry
and the wind swept them up
to build the clouds
in what is the first sky of summer

Celebrate with the young lambs quarters
growing in the yet untilled garden
Wilt them in garlic and oil in a cast iron pan
whip in half a dozen eggs,
dot with hearts of artichoke
and goat cheese coins
When the eggs are just set
slide under a hot broiler for a few moments only
until the frittata puffs and is beautiful
Tip it onto a board and cut into wedges for serving

The encircling forest has not the order of our wanting
yet we know it since the time
we rose on two feet and listened
to the calling birds to guide us
and read the shadows of the leaves
on the grass like books

We can look at the crystalline blue of the sky
and feel the catch of our heart –
that it belongs to the blue
    not to us

Don't look away
    look deeper – let your heart take you there
        Fear not
            the wind will hold you up
            the trees stand by you shimmering
            the birds' simple song show you how

Carrots and Peas

MAKES 4 SERVINGS

4 carrots, cut on the diagonal into ¼-inch slices
1 cup peas, shelled
1 tablespoon olive oil
½ cup sweet onion cut into ½-inch dice
½-inch length ginger root, finely grated
Salt and freshly ground pepper

Place carrots in steamer basket in a pan with 2 cups
salted water. Make sure the water does not submerge
the bottom of the basket. Steam until the carrots
brighten and are just tender to the point of a knife,
about 5 minutes. Drain.

Heat olive oil in medium sauté pan. Add onions
and peas. Cook over medium heat until onion is
translucent. Add carrots and stir. Add the ginger. Season
with salt and pepper to taste.
Serve.

HUMILITY

The wild carrot is in bloom
the long stems balance
the flowers like so many plates
   tatted doilies for offsetting
     sunshine

Below them the blue coins of chicory
wink like christmas lights
a mass of yellow flowers beams beneath,
telegraphing their fragrance
   their live-ness

If you can find your way
to lie down in a field
of flowers like these
you can get a hint of
   how they live

It's crowded
scores of different plants
assert themselves
   without straining
and while they spiral up and out
it's more to greet the sun than to grasp it

Tomorrow has no currency
the sun is in the sky
   now the bees, ants and butterflies
ride the rays down to the blooms
work without toil
and set to the matter-of-fact
business of life

Happiness vibrates from here
   you can feel it

In the heat of the year
carrots are cooling and delicious
scrub them and slice them at an angle
into thin disks, pair them with sweet onion
and snap or snow peas
steam the carrots briefly in salted water
while you heat olive oil in a broad pan
cook wedges of onion and peas together
not long at all
add the barely soft carrots
and a good grating of fresh ginger, salt
stir and cook another minute or two
everything will be still crisp
full of individual flavor

Each plant bores into the black earth
   just as it elevates itself into the open air
Enthralled with its one life
it grows by the wayside as a weed

Figs

16 fresh figs (Fresh figs yield to pressure, but do not
    drip syrup.)
¼ pound Gorgonzola cheese
1/3 cup walnut halves, toasted
Basil leaves for wrapping
Balsamic vinegar for dipping

Arrange ingredients on a platter in small bowls and
plates as necessary. Serve.

VIRTUE

These nights are the best piece
   of summer
The temperate air is an extension
   of our breath
      and seems not to move
The languid trees, the sky,
and the moon in her veil of clouds
   are as still as a painting
and one wonders if our antics
on the grass — our ball play, our cartwheels,
our dancing delight in the night
   are but another brush stroke
      on the great canvas of summer

Now night seems even more natural
   than the day
We listen to Romeo sing his love
   under the leafy splendor of the park
We eat quietly and sip wine
   children scoot past the stage
When Juliet thrusts the dagger
   into her own breast
the squeak of the playground swing
   keeps rhythmic, mournful time

Each day the night retreats
   into the shadows of the trees
we reach up into the leafy skirts
   of their branches
      and bring down their fruits

The figs can scarcely keep their hold on the trees
   the syrup hangs from them
      in a surfeit of sweetness

They need no preparation —
     we take one into our mouths
        and it comes to us — the vivid pleasure
           of our first food

Although we have no memory of it
     it is written in our body
     how we took our mother's soft teat
     into our mouths and drank in life
     Next to our breath it was our first act
     and it imprinted pleasure, satisfaction,
     gratitude and love into our being
           forever more

     You can see it —
        that though everyone dotes on the baby,
     it is the mother who is special
        for she alone carries this sacred nectar
     the one we spend our life long–
        –ing for

We pick the figs carefully
     and place them on a plate
There is cheese and wine
     and other things
but the figs are the sacrament
     we share in the candlelit night
they are the goodness of life
     They are virtue itself

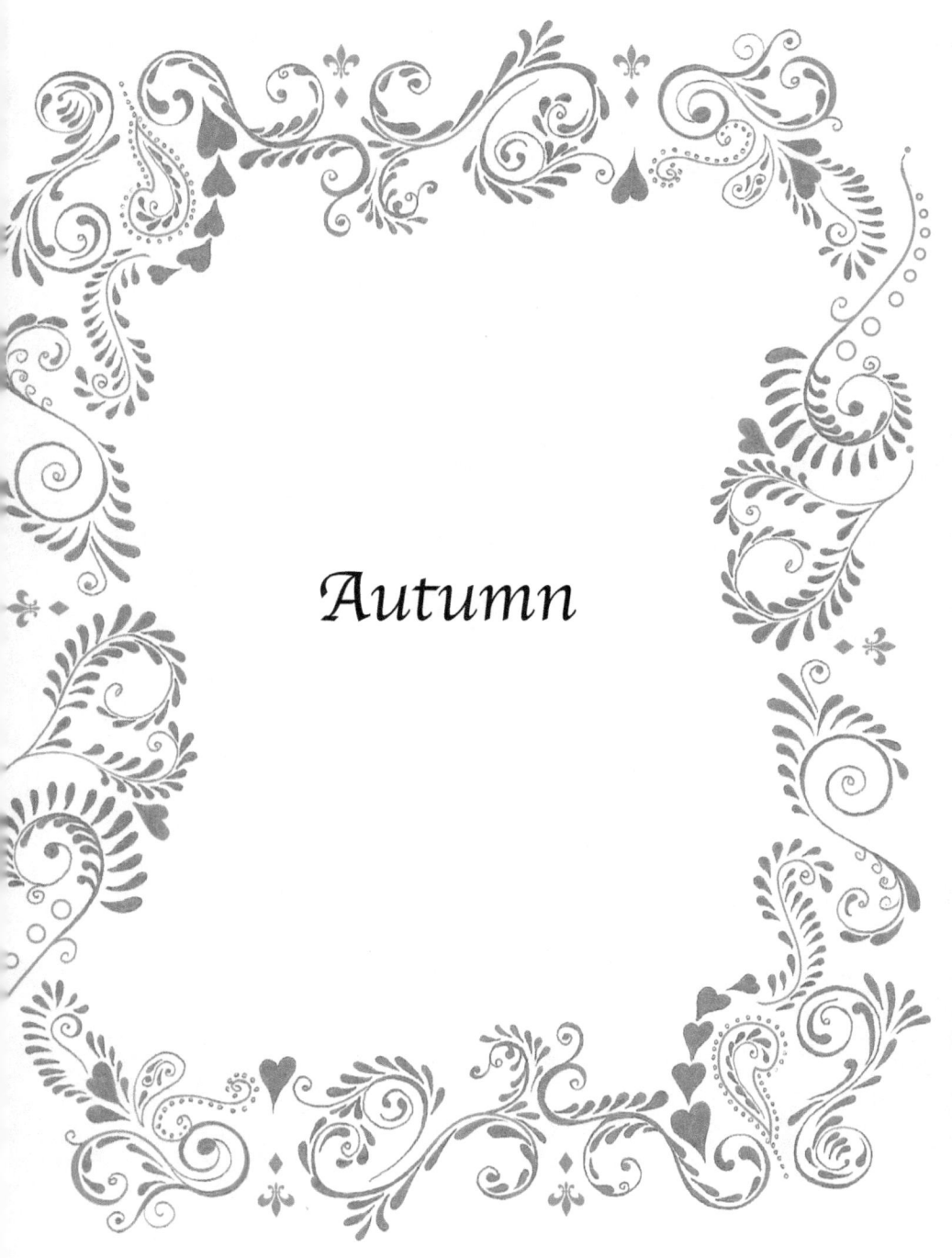

Autumn

Tagliatelle With Mushrooms

MAKES 4 SERVINGS

1 pound tagliatelle
3 tablespoons unsalted butter
Olive oil
10 ounces fresh mushrooms, such as oysters,
    hen-of-the-woods, maitake and devil's trumpet,
    chopped fine
1 large clove garlic, minced
Salt and freshly ground pepper
1 ounce cognac
1/3 cup heavy cream
¼ cup parsley, minced

Bring 4 quarts of salted water to a boil. Add tagliatelle.
Stir well. Cook pasta until al dente. Drain, reserving a
cup of pasta water.

Meanwhile, melt 1 tablespoon butter with 1
tablespoon olive oil in a large skillet over medium-high
heat. Add mushrooms and shake skillet to spread the
mushrooms evenly across the pan.
Season liberally. Do not stir. Allow the mushrooms to
give off their liquid, about 5 minutes.

In a separate pan melt 2 tablespoons butter. Cook until
browned lightly. Set aside.

Once the mushrooms are cooked, raise the heat to
medium heat. Pour the cognac over all. Cook until the
cognac is largely absorbed. Lower heat. Gently stir in
cream and reserved butter.

Add pasta and coat completely with the sauce. Add
pasta water until the dish is velvety. Adjust seasonings.
Serve immediately.

THE FOREST FLOOR

The sultry night air has the cicadas
thronging through the trees
sending up their song
crickets kick in with the minor notes
It gets loud on warm nights
yet provokes a calm not unlike listening
to the ocean surf

Meanwhile late summer prompts other mysteries:
mushrooms sprout on logs, lawns
in among the leaf litter
heaving rocks out of the way
toppling trees

If you are lucky enough to know
what you're doing
they are a treasure trove to bring home
and if you don't
there's always the store
Go for the season's gems: hen-of-the woods,
chanterelles, devil's trumpets, oysters and maitake

Sliced and cooked in equal measures
of butter and olive oil
a little crushed garlic, salt and lots of fresh black pepper
they make pasta fit for a carnivore
If you splash in a little cognac, cook it off
and finish with some heavy cream
you can invite company

Use a broad noodle like tagliatelle to lap it up
minced parsley for sparkle
swirl in some more browned butter
and a little of the pasta water
to make the whole thing
velvety succulent and rich

After dinner take yourself outside
and join the bugs singing in
the deepening dark
watch the stars light one by one
    then all at once

That's it! That's all there is —
    everything

Squash and Cauliflower Soup

MAKES 6 SERVINGS

2 tablespoons ghee or olive oil
1 small head cauliflower, broken into florets
1 buttercup squash, peeled and cut into 1-inch dice
2 medium yellow onions, peeled & chopped
2 medium potatoes, scrubbed and cut into 1-inch dice
2 cloves garlic, peeled & crushed
1-inch length fresh ginger root, peeled and finely grated
1 teaspoon turmeric
1 teaspoon coriander, ground
1 teaspoon cumin, ground
6 cups water or stock
Salt and freshly ground pepper to taste
½ cup cilantro, minced
Whole milk yogurt

Heat oil in deep pot or dutch oven. Add cauliflower, squash, potatoes and onions and cook over medium heat for 10 minutes.

Add garlic, ginger, turmeric, coriander, cumin, and salt to taste. Stir and coat vegetables well with spices. Add water or stock. Bring to a simmer, cover and cook for 25-30 minutes, or until vegetables are tender. Add more salt if necessary, freshly ground pepper and cilantro.

At this point the soup may be served as is, roughly mashed with a potato masher, or pureed in batches in a food processer or food mill.

Serve with a generous dollop of yogurt.

INKLING

The afternoon is as silent as a painting
only the wind moving through the tops of the trees
betrays the life that teems there
Look and you will see the commerce of the wind:
the drift of seeds on its currents
the birds moving on in small pulsing skeins
and the weather shifting — imperceptible
except in the faint race of some forgotten
current in our veins

The next day thunder brings a deep rain
and after a month of salad days
soup suddenly appeals
onions, cauliflower, potato and squash
chopped in a spicy broth of garlic,
ginger, turmeric, coriander and cumin
tastes wonderful
When the vegetables become soft
cool it all down with some tangy yogurt
salt, pepper and a handful of fresh herbs

It feels newly satisfying
like we've never had these vegetables before
like we've been given another chance
to live deeper, see farther, love a little more

Next thing you know you've stayed up later
than you should but long enough to see
the winnowing moon crest the horizon
and for a long moment you stare
with the rest of the stars
then head to bed and sleep
in a light that is infinitely old
and yet touching us for the very first time

Wheat Berries

MAKES 6 TO 8 SERVINGS

½ cup wheat berries
½ cup barley
½ cup wild rice
Lemon juice
I cup navy beans
I green bell pepper, chopped fine
½ cup parsley, minced
¼ cup red wine vinegar
1/3 cup olive oil
Salt and freshly ground pepper

Soak wheat berries covered in water with one teaspoon of lemon juice 4 hours or overnight. Drain and rinse well. Repeat the same process for the barley and wild rice in separate bowls.
Soak the beans covered in 3 cups water 4 hours or overnight. Drain and rinse well.

Bring 1 ½ cups salted water to a boil in a small pan. Add wheat berries. Reduce heat, cover and cook 45 minutes or until grain is tender and water is absorbed.

Repeat same cooking process for barley and rice, cooking each in separate pans.

Bring 3 cups water to a boil. Add beans. Reduce heat to low, cover and cook beans about 35-45 minutes or until beans are just tender.

Allow grains and beans to cool. Mix together in a large bowl with pepper, parsley, vinegar, olive oil, salt and pepper. Mix well. Adjust seasonings.

Allow to sit one hour before serving.

THE UNDERSIDE OF DESOLATION

The railroad tracks are studded with weeds
here the plants grow unimpeded
they come to these deeply disturbed places
    and grow undisturbed by mowers, sprays or foot traffic

Dig in the soil they're in
you'll find it black and fragrant
glass, rocks and tar too,
but the plants know how to heal a place
and spruce it up with their lavish leaves
    redress with wily roots

The grasses have erected their seed heads
some nod in the breeze — to look at them it's impossible
    to stifle a smile
others are a fretwork of angles,
each seed the seat of another and on up
all with shiny coats that catch the slanting sunlight
billions of seeds
    that much light — concentrated
like they're generating it themselves

Wheat, barley, oats, rice —
all seeds like these capture
the sunlight and store it — how handy for us

Wheat berries simmered in salted water until tender
barley cooked the same, wild rice likewise
mixed together with cooked beans,
green pepper chopped, a generous splash of wine vinegar
olive oil, plenty of fresh ground black pepper and salt
    make a fine side dish or topping on a hearty green salad

This is how we harvest the light
take it in and in turn shine outward
    seeds of beauty — each of us

Rose Hips

MAKES 4 HALF-PINT JARS

3 cups fresh rose hips
2 cups evaporated sugar cane crystals
2 tablespoons lemon juice
½ envelope pectin

Clean rose hips by removing the dried sepals that hang from the bottom of each hip. Rinse.

Place hips in a large non-reactive pan with ½ cup water. Bring to a boil. Reduce heat and simmer for about 20 minutes or until fruit is soft.

Allow to cool. Run the fruit through a chinois, a cone-shaped sieve, to remove seeds.

Return fruit to pan over medium heat. Mix pectin and ½ cup sugar in a small bowl. Add to fruit. Bring to boil. Add remaining sugar and lemon juice. Boil for 1 minute. Remove from heat.

Fill sterilized jam jars to ½-inch below rim with fruit. Top with sterilized rings and lids. Allow to cool.

TIME

To see the yet-leaved trees
   float in their bowl of blue
      is to annihilate doubt

To gaze into the heart of the last rose
   vibrating a message
     for which there is no translation
is to know meaning

We may think we don't have time
   to converse with a rose
but that's silly —
what can time have over
the sumptuous red
   the same red that lopes though our own bodies
or the extravagant delicacy of its petals
   the breath of its perfume

Time is a simple convenience
   but a rose embodies the Beautiful

How purely it faces us
   how yielding

and it does yield
   to black
Its petals curl
   and fall
     nameless
on the black earth

But its round shiny hip stays behind
   to bob in the blue
      fattening rouging ripening its seed
red spotlights in the clutter
   of a yellowing bramble
Until these too draw in on themselves
   shrivel and soften
      into a kind of dusky orange raisin

This is when they are ripe to pick
Pour several cups in a pan
with half as much water
Cook at a simmer until the hips
fall apart and bubble
Run them through a sieve
to extract the seeds
then stir the fruit with sugar
a little pectin and a spoon of lemon juice
Cook it down to a thick sauce
to pour over yogurt cheese
or to spread on toast

Ambrosia itself has no comparison

It's all out there
free to everyone
the blue, the rose, the shining trees
all you have to do is open the door
   and let it in

Quick, do it now
   before time
      convinces you you can't

Barley

MAKES 4 SERVINGS

1 cup hulled barley
lemon juice
½ teaspoon salt
2 tablespoons butter
Freshly ground pepper
Ume vinegar

Soak barley covered in water with one teaspoon of
lemon juice 4 hours or overnight. Drain and rinse well.
(See note.)

In a medium pan bring 3 cups water to boil. Add
barley, salt and 1 tablespoon butter. Reduce heat to
low and cover. Cook for 50 minutes to an hour or until
barley has absorbed water and become soft.

Adjust seasoning. Serve with a pat of butter and a
generous cracking of pepper. Add vinegar to taste.

NOTE: Soaking grains in water with lemon juice or
whey helps to break down the phytic acid that covers
the grain, making the nutrients in the grain more easily
absorbed.

HOSTING SUMMER

The breeze pulses through the trees
    like they're breathing in light
Behind them the sky is immaculate

Here and there the butterflies are pinned
to their namesake bushes
They fold their wings into a mudra
    and meditate for all we know

They cavort everywhere: high in the pines,
across the dunes, in and out of the shadows
Their flight is not linear — instead it threads
through the air, looping over itself,
    haphazard and effortful
Their wings seem a tad large and too heavy
to keep them aloft, yet they skid
through the air feverishly until — they stop
still as the sky behind them

This they do as the summer drains it's glass of light
then answering some unknown signal, they leave —
the moon has just begun gestating,
perhaps her fullness is their sign —
but leave they do on their clumsy and improbable wings
They launch over the great ocean
with her winds, her weather, without a stick to stand on
They will fly the nameless miles until they light
on a tropical tree where they have never before been
to congregate with their own kind
    by the millions

By then the dawn here
will frost the grass
We will want socks on our toes
and something hot to eat in the morning

Barley kernels cooked soft
with butter and salt
one part grain to
two and an half parts water
Like rice, but longer
nearly an hour
Now dash ume vinegar
over a bowl-full, maybe a bit more butter
and a crackling of good black pepper

Not the usual fare
but why the usual
when the extraordinary
is swirling ever around us
the great blue sheet billowing above
and our sated guest, this summer gone,
a kaleidoscope of butterflies riding his coattails

Baked Pumpkin

MAKES 6 SERVINGS

1 small pumpkin, cut in quarters with seeds removed
Olive oil
8 sprigs fresh thyme, stems removed
Freshly ground black pepper
Fleur de sel

Preheat oven to 375°. Place pumpkin pieces in a foil-lined baking pan. Drizzle with olive oil. Sprinkle thyme over pumpkin with salt and pepper to taste.
Bake 40 minutes or until pumpkin is fork-tender.

Wild Rice Salad

MAKES 6 SERVINGS

1 cup wild rice
2 tablespoons olive oil
1 medium-sized yellow onion, chopped fine
2 cloves garlic, minced
2 cups red cabbage, finely sliced
¼ cup tarragon, minced
¼ cup parsley, minced
¼ cup raspberry vinegar
Fleur de sel
Freshly ground black pepper
6 ounces fresh raspberries

In a small pan bring 3 cups of salted water to a boil. Add wild rice. Reduce heat to simmer and cover. Cook until kernels puff open, about 45 minutes. Drain excess liquid.

Heat olive in large sauté pan over medium heat. Add onions and garlic. Cook until translucent. Add cabbage. Cook 5 minutes more. Add cooked rice, herbs, vinegar, salt and pepper to taste. Serve with fresh raspberries.

KINGDOM COME

Have you noticed
how the sun's slanting light
makes the tall grass shine
how it sets the fall leaves alight

The winds will be here soon
setting off a blizzard of color
and finishing off the vines
to leave the pumpkins ripe and rotund

It's a small thrill to bring one in
to light up the place
But, you know, pumpkin is very good cooked
cut up in wedges
drizzled with olive oil and scattered with
the fresh thyme that grows free and rife
in enlightened lawns
a little pepper some good salt
(break out the fleur de sel)
and baked in a slow oven until tender

You can have it along side your usual fare
or put it front and center and make a salad
of wild rice and herbs and red cabbage
while it's in the oven

Eat outside one last time
sit like royalty on a wool blanket in the gold grass
and watch the birds flock past
the colored leaves spiraling down at your feet

Ratatouille Pie

MAKES 6 SERVINGS

1 10-inch pie crust, baked
1 large eggplant, cut into very think lengthwise slices
2 medium zucchini squash, cut into very thin
    lengthwise slices
1 pound plum tomatoes, cut into lengthwise quarters
    and seeded
2 medium yellow onions, halved lengthwise
    and thinly sliced
3 cloves garlic, thinly sliced
1 green bell pepper, halved lengthwise and thinly sliced
Olive oil
Salt and freshly ground pepper
16 whole basil leaves

Preheat oven to 375°. Lay eggplant and zucchini on
sheet pans and brush on both sides with oil. Sprinkle
with salt and pepper.

Place tomatoes, green pepper, garlic and onions in
oven proof dish. Add 1 tablespoon olive oil, salt and
pepper.

Roast vegetables for 15 minutes. Remove from oven
and cool.

Place half of tomato mixture on bottom of pie crust.
Follow with half of eggplant and half of zucchini. Lay 8
basil leaves over all. Repeat with remaining tomatoes,
eggplant and zucchini. Top with remaining basil leaves.
Drizzle with olive oil. Bake for 35 minutes.

GENUFLECTION

So you're going to have a baby
your project got accepted
you made the deposit
she said yes
he got in

The engine that drives us
past the clear light of dawn
the gentle trees and their song
past the sunset that rings
    a bell of peace
past the spiraling stars
    blinking on and off
the moonlight their path

Is the engine that can stop us
to touch our knee to the ground
as we fall forward into the heavenly grass
and breathe in the goodness
we were meant for

We spread a blanket away
    from the shade
hand around wedges of pie
made with tomatoes, eggplant
and summer squash dressed
in herbs, olive oil and parmesan cheese
someone pours wine
another slices plums

This is a song
about what it is to sit on the earth
to sing the sun warming our backs
    in a landscape of every living thing

Kale Salad

MAKES 4 SERVINGS

10 kale leaves, rinsed with stems removed
1 tablespoon fresh dill, minced
1 tablespoon fresh mint, minced
1 tablespoon fresh parsley, minced
4 cups watermelon, cut into 1-inch chunks
Coarse sea salt and freshly ground pepper

Pumpkin Seed Dressing

MAKES 1 CUP

2/3 cup olive oil
¼ cup lemon juice
¼ cup ground pepita seeds
2 teaspoons Dijon mustard
1 teaspoon honey
1 teaspoon salt
 teaspoon freshly ground pepper

Pour all dressing ingredients into a small jar with
a tight-fitting lid. Shake vigorously until completely
emulsified.

Tear kale leaves into 1-inch pieces and place in large
bowl. Add ¼ cup of dressing. Using your hands
massage the kale leaves with the dressing, adding more
dressing as needed. Continue to massage until kale
becomes translucent-looking, about 5 minutes.

Add fresh herbs. Toss.

Serve with watermelon chunks. Sprinkle with coarse
salt and pepper to taste.

EDGES

The estuarine currents bunch up
in the shifting tides
coagulating the river in curdled waves
    more form than liquid

Above, the clouds mimic the water and arrange
themselves in regular patterned scales
that calm and reassure us

The water looks dark, troubling
    vaguely dangerous

But the sky looks lighthearted, friendly

We trace the seam between these two realms:
the far edge of day, hint of night
the reach and pull of the tides
the last tentative heat of summer
    and autumn's yellow light

We can walk the line between the seasons
with a raw salad made from kale tips
and an assortment of harvest herbs:
dill, mint, parsley
and the unexpected delight of watermelon chunks
all dressed with lemon juice, olive oil, ground pumpkin seeds
a small spoon of honey, good salt and fresh ground pepper

The changing season sharpens our senses
stirs something in us –
anticipation/loss: sorrow's coin

But a sharp intake of breath alerts us:
we are witness to ever-unfolding change
let it thrill the heart
for we have hearts made to be thrilled

Chew Your Food

Bring your food to a table. Sit square in your chair,
both feet planted on the floor. Have nothing on the
table except your food and maybe a flower in a vase
of water.

Say a blessing over your food. Thank you for this food.

Take a bite of food. Chew the bite until it becomes
liquid in your mouth. Chew some more.

After you have completely swallowed that mouthful,
allow yourself to take another bite.

Continue with your meal, thoroughly chewing each
bite as above. Eat until sated. There is no need to clean
your plate.

CATCHING LIGHT

Some days all we see are the cars,
the pushing prams,
the meters and keys,
the tangle of wires,
the grates, poles and metal doors

When all we hear is the shifting
of papers, the clicking, the switches,
the idling engines, the music
not meant for anyone,
the static of the crumpled wrapper

When what we feel is the cold handle,
the streamlined device, the box,
the can, the cross-grain strap

But it is at this very point
that the singular, speechless tree
has bared one branch
while all its other leaves cling

Or the branches of the corner oak draw
themselves diagonal to everything
else around them
cutting our little grid
into a hundred random pieces
   so we can rest

Or the sky — near gray — subtly slides
to white and the sun lights as though under water

Or the very young girl in her plaid coat
waves goodbye
   not another thing on her mind

Or the wind blows voices
and scatters them up the street
to mingle with the leaves
each in turn spin–
    ning to the ground

Sip and drink slowly
savor what you eat
your food is fuel yes
but it is also an exchange
between you and this world:

you are
what you eat
drink see feel experience
  at this moment

Stand beneath the trees
look up into their golden boughs
the black limbs
the lucre of leaves
stand and wait a while
until one leaf falls
into your open hand

Catch this moment
in the lamplit light
  shining on
  and from within
  every
    thing

Baked Apples

MAKES 6 SERVINGS

6 baking apples, such as Empire, Rome, Stayman-
    Winesap or McIntosh, each cored and
    cut into 10-12 lengthwise wedges
3 tablespoons butter
3 tablespoons coconut crystals or brown sugar
Cinnamon
Chopped walnuts

Preheat oven to 350°. Melt butter in a large ovenproof
skillet. Add sugar and cook over medium heat until
sugar melts and butter browns. Arrange apple slices
tightly together in a spiral that fills the bottom of the
pan. Sprinkle with cinnamon.

Cover with aluminum foil. Bake for 25-30 minutes.
Serve with chopped walnuts if desired.

LOOKING GLASS

There is still time
to count shooting stars
in the open air
before the weather turns

Make some kind of fire
a few logs in a pit, some lanterns,
a cluster of candles will do
leave the music and hullabaloo inside
and listens to what's left of the cicadas,
the owl's "Who cooked the books?"
or the purr of the kitty in your lap

The breeze draws a gauze across the moon
    framing her for our delectation
Why else would there be so much beauty
    if we aren't there to celebrate it?

We took beauty and gave it a name
Before people it was light from the stars
We came along and called it,
    "wormholes in the great cloak of the sun"

    Beauty is meant for us
        and we are meant for Beauty
    We recognize it, we give it a name
        and it guides us to our true nature

Take your children lightly
under the night sky
Hold this mirror before them
so they can see the wonder
    of what they are

You may have to give them
    something to eat
all of us children love to eat
    something sweet
Quarter-sawn apples
arranged in a flower
and baked with butter and cinnamon
are friendly and can always
be spread with jam while they're still hot

Any food eaten outside by a fire is delicious
Piling together under a blanket
    is just as sweet
shining light
    back into the black

Gratitude

We sit in gratitude for the light
that moves the air
that cools the waters
that brings the rain
that wets the earth
that grows the plants
that feeds our bodies

that we may receive the light
and know peace

THANKSGIVING

This business of Thanksgiving
we learn as the obedient children we are
for every good thing we receive —
great or small — we bow our heads
our food, our family, our freedoms

Yes, all of that
   obvious and absolute

But what of the dread cold
   the bitter night
What of the loneliness
   the want not met
the loss, the ache, the tedium?

What about the bills, the bother, the b.s.!
What about this?
What about that?!

Now we can learn gratitude
and kiss every bill
embrace every aggravation
bow to bless each loss
and yes, love every enemy

This is gratitude
This is Thanks-giving

Be grateful for it all
This is what the human animal is for:
to be thankful
   to be blessed

Onion and Olive Galette
MAKES 6 TO 8 SERVINGS

Crust
2½ cups unbleached flour
2 sticks unsalted butter, cut into pieces
1 egg yolk
5-6 tablespoons ice water

In the bowl of food processor, pulse flour and butter until mixture has the consistency of coarse cornmeal. Beat the egg yolk with 2 tablespoons ice water. Drizzle into processor while pulsing. Continue to add water a tablespoon at a time, pulsing all the while until dough just comes together,

Turn into a sheet of plastic wrap. Wrap and form into a rectangular disk. Refrigerator for at least one hours.

Filling
5 yellow onions, halved and thinly sliced
2 teaspoons sugar
3 tablespoons olive oil
¼ cup Moroccan oil-cured olives, pitted and halved
1tablespoon fresh rosemary leaves, minced
Salt and freshly ground pepper

Heat olive oil in a large skillet over medium heat. Add onions and cook until translucent. Stir in sugar and continue to cook until onions have caramelized, about 30 minutes. Add olives, rosemary, salt and pepper to taste.

Preheat oven to 400°. Roll out pastry dough on a lightly floured surface until about 16 by 18-inch rectangle. Moved to a parchment lined sheet pan. Fold over edges to form a 1-inch border. Add onion mixture in even layer. Bake for 10 minutes. Reduce heat to 400° and bake for 20 minutes longer.

THANKSGIVING WITHOUT TURKEY

Turkeys fly you know
they glide out of the trees in the early morning
and scratch through the bone yard of fallen leaves
uncovering morsels
they peer over the high grass and step ever watchful
into a clearing where they feed sedate and serious
until some silent signal sets them
in a flurry back into the forest — gone

I say spare the main course
and give thanks from the side:
fresh figs filled with gorgonzola and warmed through,
caramelized onion, oil-cured olive
and rosemary galette,
buckwheat crepes laid with lox,
dill and crème fraiche
and this:
chanterelle, cranberry bean, corn and shallot
succotash along side a kabocha soufflé

Cooking in your kitchen is both a creative act and
one of love — go ahead
gather your herbs, roll up your sleeves,
pull out the stops
bring all your favorite people and food together
and remember who you are:
another animal who loves to eat
happy dining

Adzuki Beans
MAKES 8 SERVINGS

1½ cups dried adzuki beans, soaked overnight,
    drained and rinsed
1 cup quinoa, soaked overnight, drained and rinsed
Salt
1/3 cup olive oil
¼ cup lime juice
6-8 cloves garlic, minced
2 teaspoons ground cumin
1 bunch cilantro with stems removed, minced
Salt
Freshly ground black pepper

Bring 6 cups water to a boil in a medium pan. Add adzuki beans. Reduce heat, cover and simmer for 45 minutes until the beans are tender, but still hold their shape. Cool.

Bring 1 3/4 cup salted water to a boil. Add quinoa. Reduce heat, cover and simmer for 20 minutes or until liquid has been absorbed. Cool.

Mix beans and quinoa in a large bowl. Add remaining ingredients, stirring thoroughly. Adjust seasonings. Allow to sit at room temperature for 30 minutes before serving.

20/20

The yellow line of the road
the tawny awnings
the litter of leaves
all reflect the light of late morning
    cresting the treetops
        and delivering itself in an umbra
            so that we can see with our eyes
what we carry in our own heart
see how the light pierces the trees
    and our own recognition

The wind makes the light flash
blinding us pleasantly
and when we come indoors
the light continues to spark about us
enlivening the humdrum
flicking open the possibilities

How about we cook up some quinoa
and aduki beans tender
make a dressing of cilantro
garlic, salt and pepper
did I say garlic?
and lime juice
This comes from Jen
but it so rang my bell
that I had to pass it on

Connect with yourself
if the light seems too bright
surrender to it
    own it
        it is who you are

Vinegar
MAKES 1 QUART

1 quart red wine vinegar
1 tablespoon balsamic vinegar
Fallen maple leaves, clean, fresh, not yet dry and brittle

Sterilize a glass quart-sized jar in boiling water, as well as the lid.

Pack the jar with the maple leaves. Pour the vinegars over all, leaving ½-inch of space at the top of the jar. Use a chopstick to poke through the mixture to release trapped bubbles of air. Secure lid.

Allow the vinegar to rest 4 to 6 weeks. Decant the vinegar through a fine sieve into a clean jar. Keeps indefinitely.

TO BE SMALL

The leaves have called in the wind
fallen leaves boil up on the sidewalk
like hot fat in a frying pan

This one skitters sideways across the path
    for all the world
a crab chasing the surf

More leaves swoop up overhead
starting the pigeons off their perch and
the two fly together flashing and falling
writing across the clotted gray sky
a script — incomprehensible —
    yet we recognize the stir in our heart

The leaves work is not done:
they pile up and fill the air
with their winey scent
birds and small animals scratch
through them looking for bugs
that hide in their warmth

It will rain and snow
freeze and thaw
    again and again
The leaves will become the anonymous
chaff of trees: duff
    hard to be less than that
And as it is with small things
    the smallest things
exert tremendous power —
    leaves become soil

The soil feeds
  the trees

What more do we want?
Press a leaf into a book
With a handful more fill a jar
then fill that jar again with live vinegar
Seal the jar and wait
a fat month or more — the longer it sets
the more winey and sweet it becomes —
Decant the vinegar
and inoculate yourself
  against the sting of winter

Gather your leaves
not into a bag, but around your trees
line a platter with the prettiest ones
  and exalt your turkey

Leaves lavish this world with life
  gift upon gift
    We live ever in abundance

Blessing

May you exalt yourself
with every thought
with every word
with every action

May the animals come to you without fear
May the children know your name

May you help every stranger
May you be a helpmeet to your partner
May your children walk in peace

May your life be bathed in kindness
May you rest in sleep

TOAST

The rising sun streams through the streets
igniting a nimbus in the hair of passersby
It baths the face of each house
and from a distance the houses look
like so many candles aflame
in a congregation of trees

The trees themselves seem to reflect
back this light in their improbable crowns of color

At this moment, with the earth turned just so,
it's easy to recognize what's holy in each and every thing
Yet, with so much work to do, it's possible to overlook
    this gorgeous life

Work hard, be great,
    but bow before the flowers
keep the company of trees
walk in proximity of weeds
seek out the children
    and before you eat
        make a toast to the food

Extend a blessing to what you eat
and the blessing will flower
in everyone who eats it
as laughter, love and shining light

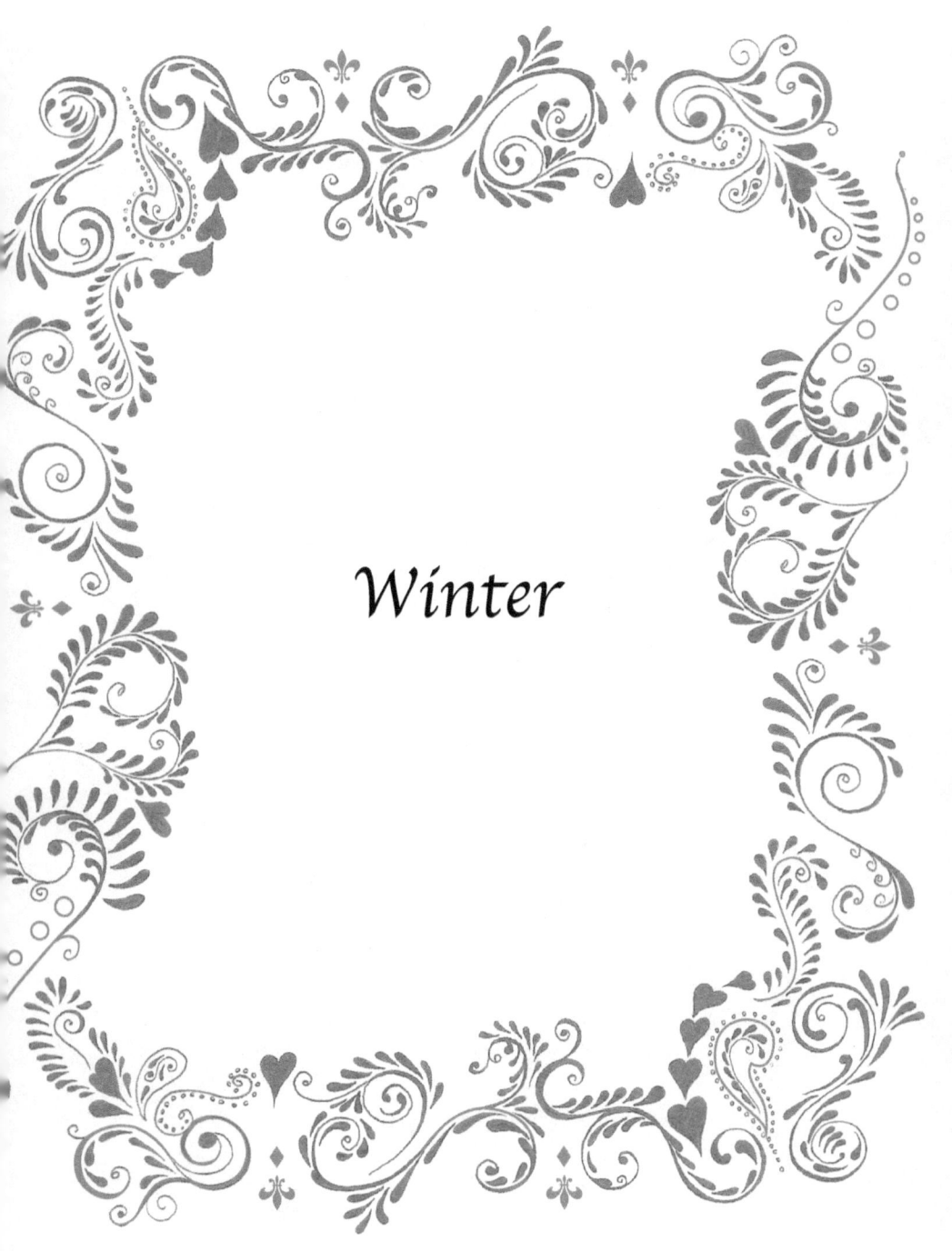

Winter

Miso Soup
MAKES 4 SERVINGS

2-inch length kombu seaweed
3 tablespoons bonito flakes (optional)
1 carrot, scrubbed, trimmed and julienned
1 3-inch length of daikon radish, scrubbed,
      trimmed and julienned
3 shiitakes mushrooms, stems removed, thinly sliced
1 frond wakame seaweed, crumbled
1 cup firm silken tofu, cut into ½-inch cubes
1/3 cup red miso paste
3 scallions, green part only, thinly sliced

In a medium saucepan, bring 6 cups of water to a simmer with the kombu over medium heat. Cook at a simmer for 10 minutes. Remove the kombu. Bring the liquid to a boil, add the bonito flakes and immediately remove from heat. Allow the broth to sit for 2 minutes. Strain through a fine mesh sieve. Discard the bonito flakes.

Bring broth to a simmer over medium heat. Ladle ½ cup of the liquid into a heat proof cup. Reserve.

Add carrot, daikon, shiitakes and wakame to the broth over medium heat. Cook for 3 minutes. Add tofu and cook gently for another minute.

Stir miso paste into reserved hot liquid to make a thick gravy. Gradually add the gravy to the soup, stirring all the while. Cook gently another minute. Do not boil.

Serve immediately with scallion greens.

HIBERNATING

See how the clouds bulge from behind the buildings
    as if on reconnaissance
next time you look they're gone
leaving an icy blue
but no more warmth
    farther in the distance light and shadow converge
smudging all the detail
there simply isn't enough light to raise the horizon
    and it's the most you'll see all day

Time for some soup:
carrot, daikon and shiitake cut into matchsticks
a finger of kombu and some crumbled wakame
simmer gently in a quart of water
until the vegetables are tender
plop in a handful of cubed tofu and cook a bit more

With some of the broth in a cup
stir in a fat knob of miso
until you have a creamy sauce
swirl into the soup and heat through,
but don't cook
ladle into bowls
flick in some minced scallion

That's it
    make like a bear
and focus in
    Spring will be here before you know it

Sweet Potato

MAKES 1 SERVING

1 sweet potato, scrubbed
1 tablespoon butter
1 tablespoon peanut butter
Coarse sea salt

Preheat oven to 375°. Rub potato with small amount of butter. Pierce skin with a fork a couple of times. Wrap in aluminum foil. Bake for 45 minutes or until a fork easily penetrates to the center of the potato.

To serve slice the potato open lengthwise. Add butters and salt to taste.

FROM HERE TO THERE

The moment you step out the front door
the wind rushes and still more leaves sift down
to skitter at your feet

Frost has limned the ground
when you look closely you see
the tiny crystals tufting the leaves —
fastidious and delicate —
  they've likely finished off most gardens

A neighbor scraping his windshield waves hello
a defunct pumpkin sits on a pedestal
falling in on itself, ghoulish at last
the air smells spicy, clean and vital

Such banal beauty is fearsome
which is probably why we tend to ignore it
it's scary to be open to that much happiness

By the time you come in
the sweet potato you put to bake is done
slice it open and smear it with a fat pat of butter
or some olive oil or both
peanut butter is good as are hemp seeds
go for it — it's a long way to lunch

Eat it outside on the top step and watch
the sun finally lift above the ridge
of buildings making the grass glisten
and the oak leaves shine

Yogi Tea

MAKES 2 QUARTS

5 cinnamon sticks
1 tablespoon cardamon pods, cracked
2 teaspoons black peppercorns
1 teaspoon whole cloves
2-inch length ginger root, peeled and thinly sliced

Place all the ingredients in a large pot with 2 quarts
of water. Bring to a simmer over low heat. Lower heat
until surface of water wrinkles, but does not bubble.
Maintain for 30 minutes. Allow to sit for 1 hour or
overnight.

Strain through a fine sieve into a glass jar. Refrigerate
for up to 1 week.

To serve heat 1 part tea to 1 part milk. Sweeten with
honey if desired.

DUSK

Now is the time of the crow —
    they patrol the leafless trees
with their barking calls
gracing our humdrum lives
    with a fearsome mystery

With all the leaves down
    nests are laid bare
This one holds fast in a spiny red-berried bush
the outer cup interwoven with plastic strips,
cigarette wrappers and anonymous bits of light metal
Inside twigs, pine needles and grass form a hollow
wonderfully snug and muscular
    for so tender a place

The clouds hunker down
enumerating the spectrum of gray and purple
at the horizon blotches of orange
make it seem later than it is
time to go in — the lamp is already lit

A warming tea is just the thing:
cracked cardamon pods, peppercorns, cloves,
cinnamon and a fat knob of ginger root sliced thin
Heat in water, but do not boil. Maintain 30 minutes
Come teatime, heat one part of this with one part milk,
add nectar or honey to sweeten

Gather yourself into your nest,
be like a bird — completely present
Feel the beauty vibrate inside and out

The crows swoop past
one perches in a long-dead pine
    it flaps its black silk wings
and settles in to call in the night

Golden Milk

MAKES 1 CUP

¼ cup turmeric powder
½ teaspoon freshly ground black pepper
1 cup milk
½ teaspoon ginger root, peeled and finely grated
½ teaspoon honey

Place turmeric powder and pepper in small saucepan with ½ cup water. Cook, stirring constantly, over medium-high heat until a thick paste is made. Remove from heat. To store refrigerate paste in a lidded jar.

In a small pan heat milk with ½ teaspoon turmeric paste, ginger root and honey. Stir. Serve immediately.

POSSIBILITY

Here it is
the blue light of morning
the last of the moon-fed night

What's left of the maple's leaves
out back radiate a buttery yellow
they are not leaves so much
as shapes of color perfectly aligned
with the tender blue breath of morning

> Out of the blackness
> the world takes form
> darkness giving shape to the light

The night silent as smoke
slips the sheets from the bed of sleep
color and movement arise
as we rise from dreamless sleep
to create
  what we are

While we sleep we can inoculate ourselves
against besetting infections with a cup of milk
warmed with turmeric, ginger and honey
Drink it warm and you will sleep sound
and awake strengthened

Each night takes us
to the fount of nothingness
so that we may be revealed
to ourselves in the light of day
and make manifest
something never before
exactly
    like
       this

A new chance from the plenitude
of possibility to be
a beating heart
  a breath
    in the space
    where nothing
      was before

Compost

To make garden compost begin with several shovelfuls of soil. Add a grocery bag full of dried fallen leaves. Add one bucket of kitchen scraps, including potato peels, banana skins, root ends, bruises, dings and discolorations from fruit and vegetables. Exclude meat and bones, but shrimps shells and the occasional lobster shell is permissible.

Cover the kitchen scraps with more leaves and another shovelful of soil.

Proceed in this manner for the first 5 buckets of kitchen scraps. With a garden fork, turn the compost thoroughly. It should have the moisture of a damp sponge. If it is dry, douse it with a bit of water. If the compost becomes too wet, add more leaves and turn the compost thoroughly. The compost should smell like nothing more than rich earth.

Once the compost is established you may omit the soil and leaves. Continue to turn the compost weekly, checking for the appropriate moisture level.

The occasional addition of grass trimmings, garden debris or cow manure will help to heat the compost.

In the spring and fall, remove the top layer of non-decomposed compost. Take the bottom layer that has turned to soil and use it to dress your garden, working it lightly into the soil.

FROM THE HOOP

Written by my nine-year-old daughter, Ella,
and I am very pleased to bring it to you here:

    Winter's light is a moose trailing down a path
    getting closer and closer to you
    with sparkling light floating up into the air

    Winter's light is a cup of hot chocolate
    with the steam spiraling out
    the smell coming from it
    fills the room

    Winter's light is a miracle
    from the guardian of the light:

    The season
      This season is Winter

Presented by my sister, Rita

    Compost before you compost:
    Put your kitchen scraps — those odd bits
    of cabbage, the wrinkled potato, the tough leek leaves,
    the carrot trimmings, the celery tops, the squash rinds –
    what-have-you — in a pot with water
    salt, pepper and herbs and simmer covered to make stock

    This stock can be used to cook rice, deglaze a pan,
    start soup, thin gravy, braise vegetables
    It's uses are endless, mineral-packed and flavorful
    Now your trimmings will compost all the quicker

Take this year you've lived
pull it close, thank it
and kiss it farewell
    compost indeed

Soba Noodle Soup

MAKES 4 SERVINGS

1 8.8-ounce package soba noodles
1 2-inch length kombu seaweed
½ cup cabbage, shredded
¼ cup carrot, julienned
¼ cup daikon radish, julienned
2 shiitake mushrooms, thinly sliced
½ cup mustard greens, chopped fine
1-inch length ginger root, peeled and grated
2 tablespoons cilantro, minced
2 tablespoons tamari sauce
1 teaspoon toasted sesame oil
1 teaspoon hot pepper sesame oil (optional)
2 tablespoons scallion greens, minced

Cook soba noodles according to package instructions, rinse, drain and set aside.

In a large pot bring 6 cups of salted water to a boil. Add kombu, cabbage, carrot, daikon, mushrooms, ginger and greens. Reduce heat to low and simmer for 5 minutes. Remove kombu.

Add noodles to pot with remaining ingredients. Heat through. Serve immediately.

NEW YEARS

Well here we are
    another year
and the grass is still green
there is parsley and kale in the garden
here and there a pansy blossom
steps up and bows

Take it in with what grace you can
ice will have it all and soon
and we will be reduced to noodles
    and broth

Not a bad prospect if you use soba noodles
throw in some shredded cabbage and mushrooms
a little fresh ginger
finish it with minced scallion
and a splash of tamari to pull it all together

Use what you have on hand:
carrots, daikon, cayenne and cilantro
onions, miso and fresh cubed fish
squash, sesame oil and bitter greens
poach what you want to cook
the rest can be added to the steaming bowl

See the possibilities:
breathe in and take stock
breathe out and smile
the new year awaits you
    with open arms

Kimchi

MAKES 2 QUARTS

1 large Napa cabbage, cored, quartered lengthwise and
    sliced into 1-inch pieces
1/3 cup coarse salt
4 scallions, using green part only, cut into 1-inch lengths
2-inch length ginger root, peeled and minced
1 cup daikon radish, julienned
2 teaspoons red pepper flakes

Place the cabbage into a large bowl, adding the salt as
you go. Toss well. Cover and let sit for 2 hours.

Rinse the cabbage in cold water. Drain.

In a large bowl combine the cabbage with the
remaining ingredients. Toss well.

Pack the cabbage into 2 sterilized quart jars. Fill two
small zip-lock bags with water and use as lids, tucking
the bags into the jars. Place the jars in a shallow baking
pan to capture any run-off from the cabbage.

Allow the kimchi to sit at room temperature for 5 to 7
days. Refrigerate to store for up to 1 month.

CAPACITY

From the unnameable shadows
the rank depths of forgotten beauty
a tree in winter towers
over a vise of buildings
each branch flowers into another
and again until the last
tight bud holds forth in the blue

Farther on a spruce rises as impossibly
visited by splayed crates and ill-used chairs
yet its top-most limbs are crowned with cones
this tree has found its perfection as surely
as it would standing in the high mountain forests

The tree knows how to be patient and wait
you can practice by making your own kimchi
a cabbage coarsely cut and covered with brine
add hot pepper flakes, minced ginger, radish
and chopped scallions
put it in a large jar, add enough brine to cover
A few days wait, maybe five, it is good to eat
and it will wait for you, if it must,
for some months in the frig

Look inside yourself
see the tree that flourishes there
see how it stands rooted and patient
continually reaching upward
letting all it needs come to it

Dinner Rolls
MAKES 18 ROLLS

5 cups unbleached flour
2 teaspoons salt
½ cup unsalted butter, softened
1 package yeast
1 egg, whisked

In a large bowl mix the flour and salt. Add the butter in small pieces. Work into the flour completely.

Dissolve the yeast in 1½ cups warm water. Add to flour and mix thoroughly. Add water a tablespoon at a time if necessary to form a ball.

Turn onto a lightly floured surface and knead the dough for 10 minutes until it is soft and very elastic.

Return to the bowl, cover with an oiled sheet of plastic wrap and allow to rise for 1½-2 hours or until the dough has doubled in size. Punch down the dough and knead briefly until the dough is once again silky and smooth.

Cut the ball in half. Cover one half. Roll the other half into a 13½" log. Cut the log into 9 equal pieces. Form into balls. Arrange in a buttered 9x9-inch pan baking pan. Allow rolls to rise one hour.

Proceed with second ball as above. At this point the pan may be wrapped and refrigerated for a day. Or frozen for up to a month. Thaw to room temperature and proceed as above.

Preheat oven to 450°. Brush rolls with egg. Bake 20 minutes. Allow rolls to rest 10 minutes before serving. using kitchen string

NOON

At noon the clouds create
   a bright opalescent light
like the inside of an eggshell

This light separates the black from the white
    with distinct clarity
creating a landscape
with its lumpen snow, forlorn cars
and bric-a-brac of trees
that would be imbibe-able if
   we could but pour it into a glass

The sun moves behind the scene
   seeping out as shadow play
for the snow casting itself aimlessly
that it may fertilize the cold
   and fall to the ground

While we wait we can bake bread
Soft butter worked into flour and salt
Add yeast dissolved in water and mix
Knead the dough to make a soft, elastic ball.
Allow to rise covered and warm
Punch down, knead some more
Roll into two logs, then small balls
Let the rolls rise. Bake.

Drink it in
let the landscape flow into your senses
reach not
   receive
as the ground receives
   the numberless flowers of snow
to make white
   out of light and stillness

Pomegranates
MAKES 2 SERVINGS

On a cutting board slice the ends off the pomegranate. With a sharp knife score the skin of the pomegranate in lengthwise lines at every quarter turn.

Over a large bowl pull the pomegranate apart in 4 sections. Turn each section inside out over the bowl. The seeds will pop free of the membranes. Continue with remaining sections, discarding the skin and membranes as you work.

Once you have freed the seeds fill the bowl with cold water. The remaining membranes will float to the top where they can be skimmed off with a sieve.

Drain seeds and pat dry. Refrigerate to store for up to five days.

What Love Is

My mother left today

She went on an airplane
to her side of the continent
If she didn't I wonder
that the whole thing would roll up on itself
like a map without her to pin it down

It's no more crazy
than all the other reasons
why we live so far from one another

In the early morning before the dawn
had quit coloring the clouds
her granddaughter hugged her goodbye
and took the walk to school in silence,
hung her coat and prepared for her day
hot tears all the while streaking
her flawless face

They played canasta by the hour
the little girl wearing cunning
as she would high heels and a hat

They baked bread
each standing on a different stool
to knead the dough
she ate the dark soft crumb
my mother ate the crust

They sorted through the paraphernalia
of an old woman's suitcase and traded jewelry
and planned the particulars of their next visit

She followed my mother from room to room
chattering and joking and bathing herself
in the light of my mother's love

It takes so much —
    that much —
  courage to hold
  your heart
  open and soft

I drove her to the airport
and back to the quiet house
peeled open a pomegranate
  for solace
and lifted the seeds
crouched under the tight skin
  each a bright red tear
and counted them as blessings

Fasting

Begin your fast with an intention: 21 days
No caffeine, no alcohol, no sugary foods
Plan as to avoid stressful situations

Upon rising drink a glass of hot water with a squeeze
of lemon juice. Drink water freely throughout the day.

Between 9 – 10 a.m. in the morning eat a hearty
breakfast that includes protein, whole grains, some fat,
a bowl of vegetables, a piece of fruit.

Before 2 p.m. in the afternoon eat your mid-day
meal. This is the main meal of the day. Follow as for
breakfast.

Before 6 o'clock in the evening eat a light meal, such as
vegetable soup and a fresh salad.

Between 6 p.m. and 9 a.m. eat nothing at all, drinking
only water.

In the evening maintain a quiet schedule of
contemplation.

Begin program with one day of this fasting routine
followed by a day of no fasting. Alternate fasting with
no fasting days for one week. For the second week, fast
daily. The third week fast on alternate days.

Consult with your physician before starting a fasting
program.

THE DARK

The black rose of winter
opens her petals unfurling darkness
   into the ever-deepening night
A black so dark it is an obliterating form
like fire — the fire of darkness
burning with a black flame
Quick to extinguish it
we strike the match
flip the switch
Still the night fingers its way
around us, smoldering in the halls
and the far corners of the garden
  blazing in the distance

   Wait
Stay a while in the dark
Let it take you up
   and drink you down
Give yourself over to this annihilating
   nothingness
Let it take you outside
   your self
that you may go deeper inside

Darkness is our cue
to recover our equanimity
to poise ourselves gently
   within ourselves
It is the place of rest, repose and restoration
It is where we give
ourselves up to the unknown
   and the unknowable

where we release our frail hold of control
and lie supine within the petals of the rose
    and dream

Sometimes eat nothing at all
    drink clear water
and forgo your meal
Thank the heavens for this one life
    for this muddle in the dark

    still and quiet

The scent of morning is well-nigh here

Rice Pudding

MAKES 2 SERVINGS

2 cups cooked rice
½ cup whole milk
¼ cup golden raisins, chopped fine
¼ teaspoon ground cinnamon
1 tablespoon ground flax seed
Sheep milk yogurt
1 tablespoon maple syrup
¼ cup raw almonds, chopped

In a small pan heat the rice and the milk over low heat. Add raisins and cinnamon. Stir gently and heat through.

Meanwhile heat a skillet over medium heat. Toast almonds for 2-3 minutes until fragrant. Set aside.

When pudding is hot remove from heat and stir in flax seeds.

Serve in bowls with a spoonful of yogurt, a drizzle of maple syrup and a topping of walnuts.

LONGING

Right around now
when the ice sheets the ground
when all our tools are cold to the touch
and the ease of living has backed away a few steps
we begin to perceive
the light stretching to fill more of the day

We wake up to more light
it follows us home a little longer
it may even invite us to watch the winter sun
rouge the low lying clouds that seem to gather
at dusk no matter how clear the day

We hunker home and yearn
for something sweet and all we have
is last night's rice

Warm it up with little milk over a low flame
add a spice: cinnamon, or ground cardamon or nutmeg
now a little fruit: maybe raisins or cranberries dried
maybe some seeds: sunflower, sesame or freshly ground flax

You're on a roll now
the kitchen smells good
the day has receded

Scoop everything into a bowl
serve with a big dollop of yogurt
drizzle maple syrup, add a few nuts

From the window you can see
the sky has given way
to the backlit blue of twilight
by the time you're done it will be black
and you will be warm, nested
and content on a winter night

Sprouts

MAKES 2 CUPS

I cup dried mung beans

Rinse beans in cold water. Place in a large bowl and soak beans in cold water for 12 hours.

Drain and rinse in cold water. Drain.

Place seeds in a colander lined with a cotton kitchen towel. Cover with a plate.

Rinse twice a day, morning and night for 3 to 5 days until sprouts are the desired length. Do not rinse before storing.

Refrigerate to store in a container with a lid.

DAY-BY-DAY

In the lamplight of late evening
sparrows congregate in the ivies
other birds swarm and chase the light
through the sky flashing their undersides
then their backs — this way and that —
Why do they do this?
It's a human question

Not much later they will have disappeared
into the trees, the eaves,
the cold dark night

Each mystery nests inside another
the sun sets and drives us homeward
another day closer to spring

We can bring it closer still by sowing
a few seeds in a jar: mung beans are classic
soak two spoonfuls overnight in a quart of water
next morning they've started to grow
drain them well and lid the jar with cheesecloth
rinse them a few times throughout the day,
drain again and you'll see their tails begin to emerge
then leaves and with a little sunlight — green
all this in a few short days of winter

Place yourself in the hoop of life
look to the left and the right of you
recognize your relatives:
the plants, the winged ones
Stand squarely on the ground
hold your head heavenward
another day done well

Bean Soup

MAKES 4 SERVINGS

1 cup cannellini beans
1 bay leaf
2 tablespoons olive oil
1 small yellow onion, cut into ½-inch dice
3 cloves garlic, minced
1 teaspoon dried marjoram
½ teaspoon dried oregano
1 carrot, cut into ½-inch dice
1 large yukon gold potato, cut into ½-inch dice
1 medium turnip, cut into ½-inch dice
½ cup celery root, peeled and cut into ½-inch dice
3 ripe plum tomatoes, cut into ½-inch dice
3 leaves kale, finely chopped
Salt and freshly ground pepper
Parmesan cheese, grated

Soak beans in water overnight. Drain. Rinse.

Place beans in medium-sized pot with 6 cups cold water and bay leaf. Bring to a boil. Lower heat and simmer until beans are al dente, about 30 minutes.

Meanwhile in a separate pot, heat olive oil over medium heat. Add onions and garlic and cook until they are translucent. Add dried herbs and stir. Add the remaining vegetables. Stir and cook for 5 minutes.

Add cooked beans to pot. Add 2 teaspoons salt and ½ teaspoon pepper. Cook for about 15 minutes or until all the vegetables are tender. Adjust seasonings.

Serve in bowls with Parmesan cheese sprinkled on top.

EXTREMITIES

The trees at sunset
are the bare trees of Rembrandt
their branches break up the roseate light
into leaf-shaped fragments
    a cathedral window
      through which the light shines

The trees themselves stand black
the world spins, yes! spins
the light becomes stronger
    the colors clearer
      as the horizon rolls away from the sun

For a few moments it's as if
we are looking through a lens
that magnifies color —
    each hue more vivid
      the light more vibrant
      amid its cherubim of clouds

In the time it takes to reel in the night
you can cook a pot of beans at the back of the stove
— nothing wrong with those from the can
but these taste very good
Cover them with an inch or two of water (and a lid)
and simmer until they are almost soft
Now add some herbs, marjoram maybe,
root vegetables — carrots, potatoes,
rutabagas or turnips, try celery root —
that gnarled medusa — some kale,
chopped tomatoes or some paste
salt and fresh pepper
and anything else that appeals

Cook it all gently
until the vegetables are tender
and the broth delectable
Serve steaming bowls of it
with grated parmesan cheese

Later, the sun subdued
    and night not yet assembled,
the snow covers the ground
    in a distinct blue
    the sky nothing short of pink

That we do not bend
before this spectacle
but blithely live within it
is its own marvelous miracle:
    we turn and turn
    in and of color and light

Oatmeal Bath

MAKES 1 BATH

2 cups rolled oats
½ cup dried lavender flowers
Coconut oil

Using kitchen string, tie up the oats and flowers into a 16-inch square of double-layer cheesecloth.

Pour a hot bath and submerge the bag all the while. Squeeze the bag frequently to release the oat milk from the oats.

When the bath is cool enough to enter, but still quite hot, submerge yourself up to your chest.

Use the bag as a cloth to wash your skin. Remain in the water for 10 minutes.

Once out of the bath, towel yourself briskly. Apply pure coconut oil to your skin.

Finish with a brief cold shower.

INTERSECTIONS

This, the fifth season, stands
in the space between winter and spring

It holds the weightless flakes of snow
that float earthward to weigh
down the fields and soak them through
so that the grass will fatten
in the morrow's warm sun

It holds the blue sky keenly
pierced by the spires at noon
the flashing buildings
every reflecting surface giving
itself up as if in applause

It holds the birds stirring in the shrubbery
the mourning dove's call:
　　　the sound cold makes in the snow
they face the sun in unison
each shining breast a beacon
then wheel together in the sparkling air
　outwitting doubt

It holds the still stand of trees
without one leaf to dress them
they sing the oldest song
the song of glory —
　of untamed perfection —
each bud pressed against the matchless cheek of sky

Let the season hold you
in a rare bath
Have the water run hot over a cloth bag
filled with oatmeal and tied

Allow the water to cool enough
for you to get in and submerge
up to your chest for 10 minutes
Squeeze the bag periodically
Think no thoughts
listen to music
   allow yourself to be happy
and emerge with soft, soothed skin

The season holds us gently
it holds our tolerance for slush and bother
for canceled plans, thwarted efforts
so that we may bow to every circumstance
   and embrace it
      as sufficient unto our need

Food

Food is the universal language. Not only for humans;
it is the language of all life:
    To live is to eat; to eat is to live.

Food allows us to take our place at the table of life.
It is our privilege for these short moments we call
years to eat the food this planet yields; to take food
into our bodies and make ourselves anew each day.

Food is the handmaiden of this one life. And it is only
when we about to die that we stop eating.

Eat. Eat well. Honor your food. It is your privilege.

THE SYCAMORE

The sycamore stands delicately at the curb
    like a woman about to enter the bath
Her naked branches sway silently
    fingering the breeze
The small globes of her seed pods dangle
    with the alluring bob of ornaments

Caught in her tresses a broken branch
    hangs poised at its awkward angle
Nothing wrong with this imperfection
    but the eye follows it to see deeper

She stands within the moment
    in a succession of moments
And in that moment a big fat blossom
    of snow tumbles through her canopy
followed by another
    then another

A whole sky full of snow
    flowers among her branches
floating softly
    amplifying the quiet

The tree accepts the snow
piling onto her branches
    at every curve and tip
As she accepted last week's ice
    tomorrow's rain

What food she has we cannot eat
    but without her we would have
        no standing
We would be paupers with no house
    to hold us
We would be naked in the cold
    and know no refuge

INDEX

www.ingramcontent.com/pod-product-compliance
Lightning Source LLC
Chambersburg PA
CBHW020916290526
45784CB00002BA/584